I0415412

CUT YOUR CALORIES...NOW!!

An Outsider's Insightful Journey through the Nutrition Trade
and Why the Nutrition Advice Industry Has Failed Us All

by

Ken Kaszak

40 Ways to Cut Calories and Maintain Satiety

Elm Leaf Park Press
Pittsburgh, Pennsylvania
U.S.A

Library of Congress Control Number 2018914068

Kenneth Kaszak
Cut Your Calories...Now!!
ISBN: 9781091187252

valuekaszak@yahoo.com

Second Printing
Printed in the United States of America

Cover Design: Andrea Djordjevic
Djordjevica263@gmail.com

Print and eBook Layout: Janeil Harricharan
blueoriontiger@hotmail.com

"We cannot solve our problems with the same thinking we used when we created them."
--Albert Einstein

CONTENTS

FOREWARD

I had a spinal fusion when I was 16 years old. A surgeon shaved bone from my hip and permanently attached my L-4 and L-5 vertebra together. A serious and dangerous operation at any age. I was bedridden for most of my junior year of high school and homeschooled. My true education came from reading books my father brought me from the library and watching classic black & white movies on the small TV my parents put near my bed.

I developed a love of movies. I would watch movies of all eras and genres into the early hours of the morning. After the last movie finished, there would be a short film titled "High Flight" and then the station would go off the air. "High Flight" was a poem written by a Canadian aviator narrated over footage of an airborne jet. Hard to believe now but there was a time when local TV stations would go dark at 3 a.m.

I recently saw a great movie I hadn't seen in a few years. It was released in 1984. The story concerns a man with a unique talent. He wants to share his talent with others but events go against him. After the first act, the movie fades out and the man fades away.

When the story resumes some years later the man still has his talent and still wants to share it with others. This time, he gets his chance. He is good at what he does and he loves doing it. Somebody asks him where he's been. His reply, "Well, I sort of got sidetracked." A romantic interest from the past resurfaces. It looks like we're in for a happy ending.

But wait. People who are not happy with the happiness of others decide to rain on this man's parade. The "haters" put obstacles in front of this man and attempt to derail him. But the man overcomes the roadblocks thrown at him and prevails. We then get an uplifting ending. Fade out.

If you're a movie person, you may have figured out I'm describing *The Natural.* My story has a correlation to that of Roy Hobbs, played by Robert Redford in the movie.

I developed a passion for the nutrition and fitness industries. As a person trained in economics—and having a similar passion for that field—I studied food and fitness the way an economist would—from the "value" approach. In addition to studying "what to eat," I also studied the financial incentives of the food industry and the non-profit groups who are given the responsibility to tell you "what to eat." From the start, I knew I was onto something unique.

The people I shared my insight with appreciated it. They had never heard anybody talk about nutrition the way I did. The years of nutrition advice we had been given, as I soon realized, were influenced by the financial incentives of food companies, trade associations and lobbyists representing those interests.

Unlike Roy Hobbs, Harriet Bird didn't shoot me with a silver bullet in a hotel room in Chicago. But I was taken out of the game for a while. Roy went away and, in a manner of speaking, so did I. When I achieved a certain level of acceptance, the next level I needed to get to was blocked. Members of the Nutrition Advice Industry (NAI) who received direct deposit every two weeks from a healthcare or non-profit employer went out of their way to stop my advance.

Like Roy Hobbs, I was "sidetracked." The movie doesn't show what happened to Roy during his time away but during my time away I grew my investment practice, I traveled, I had great romances, and I created. I lived a life.

But time—and technology—have gotten me back in the game. The things I learned about nutrition and fitness many years ago are more relevant now than they were then. You're about to read my story. I'm glad I can share my experiences and insight.

Roy Hobbs didn't express any anger toward the people who prevented him from sharing his talent. He just took advantage of the opportunity when his time came and made the best of it.

And I'm going to adopt that policy. In an odd way, I realize that the members of the NAI who blocked me also helped me. They gave me the "voice" that you're about to hear (read). There would be no book if I hadn't had to deal with the people I did. While I was trying to share what I learned about nutrition, they were interested only in protecting their paychecks.

Today's technology will allow me to update, add, append, or change parts of this work. While some of the calorie cutting ways may be amended—or added to—what will not change is my experiences with the NAI. Their "help" is appreciated.

Also—thanks to technology—you can go to YouTube and watch "High Flight." I've seen it and it brought back memories of those movies I watched and books I read (John Steinbeck was a favorite) into the wee small hours of the morning *(w/credit to Frank Sinatra)*.

I hope you enjoy—and appreciate—my journey.

KK

PROLOGUE ONE

I'm hoping some people reading this will be able to relate to my childhood food memories. Here they are:

Breakfast was either cereal, French toast, or pancakes. On some of the nights my father worked the 12 to 8 shift, he would bring home a box of doughnuts from Dudt's Bakery. Those sugar doughnuts were a great way to finish off a breakfast—or a great breakfast by themselves.

During the school year, my brothers and I would walk to school. Except for the times my mother went to work as a Kelly Girl, we would walk home at noon. After lunch, our mom would comb our hair before sending us back to school. When she was working, we had our cool lunchboxes (I had the Batman motif) with the Thermos inside to carry our sandwiches, apple, and a snack. If you dropped that Thermos one time, even from two feet off the ground, the inside would break and you would be without a Thermos until your parents replaced it. After school we either played outside or, if the weather wasn't cooperating, watched Paul Shannon's *Adventure Time* featuring Nosmo King and the Three Stooges or played board games.

We would eat dinner around my father's schedule. He had a laborer's job with the gas company, and we ate simple meat and potatoes-type of dinners. On occasion, my mother would experiment with different recipes she came across. I remember her making chicken breaded with smashed-up potato chips a few times. Fortunately, that one didn't get into the rotation. Fridays during Lent were usually fish sandwiches from the McGinnis Market. Every so often, you would hear the good news that we were having pizza for dinner. Long before pizza became a multi-billion dollar industry, it was a special treat to get pizza from Anjo's Pizzeria on Brownsville Road.

Our family dinners always started with a family prayer, done in silence. My father would break the silence by stating that the one minute we were quiet was his most peaceful moment of the day.

After dinner we either went back outside or stayed in and watched television. On the weekends and when school was out for summer, we would wake up, have breakfast and go outside to play baseball, basketball, touch football, ride our bikes, hike in the woods, work on a tree house or go to the library— sometimes all in the same day! We lived in a unique neighborhood and we literally had access to all those things. My early years were similar to living in a Norman Rockwell painting.

On the holidays that we didn't go to a relative's house, my mother would make the typical dinner for a family with Eastern European roots: borscht, pierogies, galumpkis and ham. The days after a holiday were as much a food treat as the holiday itself because my father would make his delicious ham and cabbage soup.

On Saturday evening, a big treat was to have ice cream. My favorite was to have the vanilla ice cream sit out for a while to get it soft and then crunch up pretzels to put in the bowl. One caveat: we could only have the ice cream if we shined our shoes in advance of 9:30 a.m. Mass and Sunday school at St. Albert's. We had an actual shoe shine box kept in the garage but I didn't have shining skills. I ended up with as much shoe polish on my hands as made it onto the shoes. After Sunday school, it was cheese and lettuce on a Barsotti's bun, and then outside to play whatever sport was in season.

Food was there but it wasn't THERE. Of course, I wasn't driving then and didn't see all the restaurants and restaurant signs along the highway, and I wasn't food shopping for a family but my recollection was that food was far less visible than it is today. I wasn't constantly being bombarded with food messages. There was no Food Channel, no shows on TV focusing on food preparation, no shows about food in other countries and no cooking competition shows. I didn't think about food the way I'm forced to think about it today.

Things have changed. For me and you. There is too much food now. And too many food encounters. Personally, socially, and professionally. Food is everywhere. Food marketing is ubiquitous. Many businesses use food as a way to attract clients. Food companies sponsor many of the thousands of shows on the hundreds of television channels now available. The industry has created products that make it easy to eat food almost anywhere—and we do so.

Stories told to me by people hearing or seeing others eating or drinking in church are too numerous to detail. I will share one that happened to me while preparing this manuscript. I am a bicycle rider. I have ridden my bike 100 times past a former synagogue that is an interesting piece of architecture. It is now a non-denominational church. I decided to attend a service to see what the inside looks like. There was one service per week. The inside was in less than stellar condition. It was a small congregation. How small? In addition to myself, there was one other person in attendance. There were two individuals helping the pastor deliver the service. So those on the altar outnumbered those in the pew.

It was a lively, inspirational service. The pastor and his helpers weren't affected by the lack of attendance. They were passionate in their belief. Halfway through the 90-minute service, I heard the unmistakable sound of a potato chip crunch. I looked over and saw my "pew-mate" had brought a plastic bag full of potato chips and was enjoying a mid-service snack. The concept of food being brought into such places has long been erased from the concept of "proper" in our society so I wasn't surprised. The fact there were only two participants in the congregation made the potato chip episode a bit more memorable.

PROLOGUE TWO

This is where the story really starts:

I found myself working in Gainesville, Florida in January of 1991. I was there on a real estate/banking assignment. A big happening going on at the time was the closing of a bar called Dub's Place. There was a movement underway to have the spot reopened. A local named Tom Petty had been the leader of the house band there until he went on to bigger things. One night, in a different bar (where many good stories have their beginnings), I met a young woman studying gerontology at the University of Florida. I was so interested in what she was studying that I decided to learn what I could about the subjects of nutrition and fitness when I returned to Pittsburgh. I set up a small "classroom" on the back porch. I was living with my father at the time. One of the reasons I wanted to learn about these subjects was the fact that my mother had passed away three years earlier from a type of cancer known as liposarcoma. Part of my thought process was that if I learned about nutrition, fitness, lifestyle factors, etc., and could convey that information to others, that maybe somebody else's mother wouldn't have to die far too young.

If the internet existed at the time, I didn't have it. My self-study program consisted of checking out nutrition books from the library, subscribing to newsletters such as the *University of California at Berkeley Wellness Newsletter* and *Tufts Health & Nutrition Letter,* and attending seminars sponsored by local healthcare providers. I also had a short-lived but insightful relationship with two local dietitians. I called, introduced myself, and explained I was applying the techniques of economic analysis and investment research to the area of nutrition. I asked if I could phone them on occasion and ask them questions related to my research. I told them I would have the questions phrased in such a way that a "Yes" or "No" answer could be given and that I wouldn't take up much of their time. This worked well, but only for a short period. I had a few conversations with these individuals, they answered my questions but, after a couple of months, they stopped calling back.

One of my fondest memories of this period was sitting on the back porch after dinner, reading my books and journals, rereading some of the books and journals when the material was a bit too complicated for me to digest, and filling my notebooks. But at ten o'clock, I put a bookmark in whatever I was reading. There was a local public television station, WQEX (Channel 16), that would play the television series *St. Elsewhere* commercial-free each night at ten o'clock. This was a groundbreaking series, not just for the quality of the writing and subplots, but for the actors who were on this show. Some of the actors you may know from other venues: David Morse, William Daniels, Ed Begley, Jr., Howie Mandel, Denzel Washington, Alfre Woodard and Cindy Pickett (who I developed a huge crush on). The series finale of this show was one of the most memorable series sendoffs of all time.

The second part of my self-study had me taking a job selling exercise equipment. I wanted to learn about exercise and figured the best way I could do it was to sell the equipment used in the process. The owner of the company I went to work for was a great guy. He gave me time to learn about the equipment, the quality of the materials used in the production, the purpose and function of each piece, and why our products were superior to the equipment found in typical sporting goods stores.

I learned the equipment inside and out. But when it came time to sell, I struggled. I found myself talking to and over potential customers only to have them walk out of the store after saying the absolute worst thing you can say to a person working in retail: "I'll be back."

There was a point where I was worried that I would be losing my part-time job. We were selling $2,000 treadmills and $3,000 home gym units—in 1992. I wasn't getting any numbers. But I can remember the exact moment when things changed for me. It was a weekday afternoon and there was a fellow named Mark in the store. He was interested in a top of the line treadmill made by a company named True. I was with him for a long time explaining the quality of the bed, the belt, the motor and the "friction coefficient." I turned him off to the $400 Sears treadmill he knew he could buy. I had been in this situation before. When I asked the potential customer if they wanted to buy the treadmill, the reply I received was "I'll let you know," or "I'll think about it," or the dreaded "I'll be back" *(funny thing is that they never came back!)*

But Mark was right there in "closing range." I could sense it. He wanted to buy. I had done a thorough job of explaining the True treadmill. The price tag wasn't an issue. He was staring at the machine.

And then I had an idea. I asked Mark, "I can have it delivered and set up Wednesday or Friday. What's a better day for you?" In the same way I phrased my nutrition questions so that the dietitians could answer with a one-word answer, I didn't give Mark the chance to say "No." His reply to me: "Friday."

And it was on. I sold more True treadmills, Pacific Fitness home gym units, Precor ski machines, steppers, stationary bikes and recumbent bikes than I can remember. I sold expensive equipment over the phone, sight unseen, to people giving me credit card information. The firm I worked for also made their own benches and imported barbells and dumbbells from China. I sold literally tons of flat benches, incline benches, decline benches, 310-pound weight sets and individual dumbbells.

The third part of my self-study was my entry into the seminar circuit. A fellow I lifted weights with on occasion got an earful from me about nutrition and weight training from my unique "value" approach. He happened to be a police officer and arranged for me to do a seminar at the Pittsburgh Police Academy. I put together a presentation, wrote my notes on 4 X 6 index cards, and made my appearance at the academy.

And this is where I hit an obstacle. I knew my material front and back, I had tremendous enthusiasm to be there, and I knew I was onto something with the "no angle, only value" approach to nutrition. But I flopped at the police academy. I was nervous, uninteresting and, I can admit now, unprepared. In front of a class of rookie police officers, I committed a crime. If being boring was a criminal offense, I would have been booked, charged, and jailed all in the same place.

I limped home from that appearance. I decided that seminars were not going to be the best avenue for me and this appearance confirmed that thought. I would return to the porch and continue my reading and note taking.

A few days after my awful appearance, I received a

phone call from the chief of the Pittsburgh Fire Academy. He told me he heard that I had a done a great seminar for the police recruits and wanted to know if I would do one for his recruits. My first thought was that he was being sarcastic. My second thought was that somebody at the police academy was playing a joke on him by telling him I did a good job. Either way, I took him up on his offer and scheduled an appearance as soon as possible—so that he wouldn't find out the truth and cancel my appearance.

Before I returned to the building that housed both academies, I cut down my presentation. I focused on insightful, relevant information that was not being presented by other nutrition educators. I threw in some material that I hoped would generate a few laughs. And it did. I focused more on my back story. I had an attentive, interested audience. For how bad my presentation was for the police recruits, my presentation down the hall for the fire recruits was spot on.

I started doing seminars on a regular basis. I did seminars at businesses, non-profit groups, and hospitals. I got paid fewer times than I did but I didn't care. I was onto something. I made four radio appearances and one appearance on a cable-TV show. All the time I was doing this I was maintaining my self-study program and trying to grow my investment practice. During this time, I was presented with various opportunities. A chiropractor/nutritionist, who was on the radio weekly promoting his practice, was starting a supplement company. I was asked to be the spokesperson for the new venture. I declined. The owner of a medical billing company offered me a job. I declined. A real estate developer I knew had invested in a mobile nerve conduction testing van. A marketing job was offered to me. I declined. I met an endocrinologist who told me he was the first medical doctor to introduce the weight loss combination of "fen-phen" (fenfluramine and phentermine). He was trying to become a "TV doctor" and asked me to market his practice. I declined. I knew what my direction was and didn't want to detour.

But the fourth part of my venture hit a major roadblock. Three years after my first seminar, the traction I had gained stalled. I wasn't getting any bookings to do seminars. I would go into the human resources department of Pittsburgh corporations and try to get them to install wellness programs in their companies. On more than one occasion, I was told by a HR representative that they wanted a wellness program but they didn't want or need me to do it. Instead, they would call their personal trainers from Bally's Fitness to come in and teach the workforce about fitness and which supplements they should be using.

A black cloud came into my life and settled over me for a few short months that seemed to last for an eternity. My "value" approach to nutrition was being met with underwhelming success, I was struggling along in the investment business and my personal life was falling apart. Nothing good was going on in my life. I was forced to do something that was embarrassing, beneath my level of education and intelligence, and contrary to the "value" approach to nutrition. What did I do that was so horrific? I took a contract with a company selling bodybuilding supplements.

I knew all the products sold in this industry and the stated purpose of each. I knew there was minimal or no value to the products but I knew how to sell the scam. I worked in the basement of an old shoe store in Cheswick, Pennsylvania. This spot was about 75 minutes away from where I lived, which was a good thing. It would have been extremely embarrassing if anybody I knew saw me slouching into the old shoe store.

My mission was to sell supplements to gym owners in the Midwest part of the U.S. so they could mark them up and sell them to their members. As my experiences in the supplement industry may become their own book, I'm going to be brief here. I will provide one beautiful example to provide insight into the true workings of the industry.

I've been in and around the real estate and investment industries for a long time. Without a doubt, the supplement industry is the most "whorish" industry I've ever been associated with. Here's the perfect example: We bought supplements from a distributor who had bought them from the manufacturer. There was a profit mark-up from the manufacturer to the distributor, another one from the distributor to us, a third one from us to the gym owners, and the final one from the gym owner to the final user. Four profit mark-ups with a profit margin each time that would make street-corner drug dealers jealous. When we started having some success selling to gym owners, the manufacturers did what anybody in an industry built on deceit and scam would do—they started calling on the gym owners directly! My supplier became my competitor. No honor among thieves.

I was able to climb out of that old shoe store because I wrote an article that was published in the *Pittsburgh Business Times*. The article dealt with the importance of investors paying low fees on their assets. The *PBT* changed my title, misspelled my last name and did unnecessary editing. But the article made some noise. I increased my client base.

From that time until now, I have lived a life, developed my investment practice, written many other articles and essays, written four self-published books plus this one, was in a great romance for seven years that turned less than great in year eight and didn't make it to year nine and, most importantly, I saw a good bit of the world. I have traveled. In summary, I've been to Asia and Europe a total of 11 times, and I've been to Cuba nine times. I've seen 36 of the 37 paintings attributed to the Dutch painter Johannes Vermeer *(the 37th, "The Concert," was stolen in 1990 and its whereabouts are still a mystery. I've seen the frame it was stolen from but not the painting).* That unique journey that took me to 12 different countries and featured a private showing of a Vermeer painting inside the basement of Buckingham Palace. I also did a "WWII" journey that took me to Normandy, Bastogne (central site of Battle of the Bulge), the River Kwai in Thailand, and Iwo Jima, where I literally stood on the top of Mt. Suribachi—site of the most famous raising of a flag in history.

My Vermeer journey ended in October of 2013 with a memorable trip to Ireland, London and Scotland. I wrote an article about my experiences that was published in *The Artist's* magazine. Coming into the end of that year, I was thinking about what project I wanted to tackle next. In my office I kept a blue Wal-Mart crate that contained articles I had read in the intervening years about nutrition and fitness that I felt were relevant, insightful or advanced the cause of "value" nutrition. I also made notes on products that were scams (if you're trained to find value in a subject, you appreciate the scams connected to that subject). I spent some time going through my crate. I was happy and impressed with the amount of information I had accumulated. I created a small library out of the information in this crate. When I did seminars in the 90s, I had a handout titled "Cut Your Calories…Now!!" It was a list of 12 ways for individuals to reduce their calories. When I finished sorting through the material in my crate I realized I now had 34 ways of calorie cutting.

At this point, I'm going to present the list. Since those two bitter cold weekends early in 2014, I have added other ways to cut calories. On an ironic note, some of the original 12 didn't make the new list of 40.

As a preview to the other side of the list, I acquired valuable insights when trying to return to the nutrition trade that are equal in importance to the list. We will address that insight in Epilogue One.

The list follows. It is broken down by the Economics of Calorie Cutting, the Physical Aspects, the Mental Aspects and the Social & Media Aspects of Calorie Cutting.

This is a new way to learn about nutrition. Pay attention to what you're about to read and enjoy the result of what I've learned traveling inside the Nutrition Advice Industry.

"I don't know what it is about food your mother makes for you, especially when it's something that anyone can make—pancakes, meatloaf, tuna salad—but it carries a certain taste of memory."
                                                                    -- Mitch Albom

PART ONE: THE ECONOMICS OF CALORIE CUTTING

Number 1 Prepare for the Week Ahead

On Sunday afternoon or evening, cut up a green pepper, a red pepper, and an orange bell pepper (the MVP—Most Versatile Pepper), along with one or two types of onions (you can alternate the type weekly) and store the items in Tupperware containers. This makes meal planning easier during the week, reduces the risk of "impulse eating" and you can use the peppers & onions in omelets, pasta dishes or when you stir fry. My new favorite thing to prepare on Sunday for use during the week: pearl barley. I used to use the Quick Barley in the box but have started buying the bagged barley. I don't do this every week but do it on a consistent basis. Because the barley absorbs the water it is prepared in, a small bag results in a lot of cooked barley. You can prepare one-half of a bag and store half for future use. I soak the barley for a few hours, drain the water and put the "prepped" barley in a pan of boiling water. It only takes about 45 minutes to prepare. I used to only eat barley with tons of onions and light red kidney beans but have found a new recipe: barley with black beans, onions (can't get enough) and tomatoes. When I first heard of this mixture, I didn't think the barley and black beans would work together but they do. A great dish.

Number 2 Teach Yourself the Economics of Food

Any idea what percentage of disposable income the average American family spends on food? No? Should be common knowledge shared by the NAI (Nutrition Advice Industry). Try 9%. That statistic only has meaning when you learn that our grandparents' generation spent about 25% of their income on food. The result? Food is cheap for the typical American family, the packaged/processed food industry, and the restaurant industry. Cheap food equals cheap calories. Food costs less to us than previous generations due to a combination of improved farming methods, focused government policies, the inflow of capital to the food and restaurant industries (a factor often overlooked in such discussions), and the competitive nature of the industry. There are not extensive barriers to entry in food production. Even though there are giant food companies at the top of the food chain (apologies for the pun), there is not a great concentration in the industry. There were 91 companies with sales in excess of $1 billion in 2013. Few industries would match this statistic. Because of the lack of barriers to entry and extreme competition, new entrants can enter the industry with minimal capital investment and start vying for share from existing industry participants.

Here is a summary of various industry players and economic factors that should make you a better user of their product:

Supermarket industry—I've been to third world countries. When I'm in a supermarket in the U.S. I often think how the poor people I've met in countries where food is difficult to come by would react if they walked into a U.S. food store. There would be fainting in every aisle in the store, plus the produce section. We have an overabundance of food. Here are some relevant statistics about the U.S. supermarket industry:

- There are between 10,000 and 14,000 new products introduced each year. Most disappear after failing to gain traction;my feeling is that the established companies introduce so many products because their margins are so high on established staples that they can take advantage of the American shoppers' desire for "new and improved" products and impulse buying.
- Some supermarkets receive more revenue from selling or leasing the most attractive shelf space to food companies than from product sales. The giant food companies are permanently parked on the shelves that they want.
- The "endcaps" in the store are responsible for generating approximately 30% of food sales. Endcaps are perfect for impulse items, "2 for 1" sales, introductory items, and discontinued items.

How does this information help you cut calories? This is knowledge you probably didn't have before. When shopping, understand that you are in a historically unique time—a period of food overabundance. Understand that the food companies, with their advertisements and package claims, are not there for your benefit. They're there for the benefit of the shareholders, executives, and employees of the company. All publicly-traded food companies have the same mission: increase shareholder value. They do this by increasing revenue, taking share from other food companies, and (something you don't see) decreasing operating costs.

Before continuing, I want to share this: I have absolutely zero problem with the way the processed/packaged food industry is structured and operates in the U.S. or with the multinationals that sell their products in the states. I am in the investment business. I believe in the structure of capitalism (or, to be more exact, regulated capitalism). I believe in companies using pre-tax revenue to invest in research and development for new products. Because they are doing these things as a corporate entity, it doesn't mean you have to follow their thread and walk into a supermarket with your impulse control turned off and load your shopping cart with every new product that catches your eye. I also don't object to the companies that sell high/empty calorie food, produced with excessive amounts of sugar/salt/fat, also producing "low-calorie" versions of the same product. They're making money on both sides of the aisle but guess what? These companies are not responsible for the obesity/Type II diabetes issues in America. We are. We are just consuming too much of their product. Regular or low-calorie. As it turns out, the processed/packaged food industry is responsible for one of the greatest developments in food history: flash frozen vegetables. This is a product that should be a major component of any household. If you think, incorrectly, that fresh produce, or produce labeled "organic" (which still may have used pesticides) is your best bet for vegetables, think again. According to the American Council on Science and Health, the highest risk of foodborne illness comes from produce and not animal protein. Flash frozen vegetables eliminate the amount of human handling the vegetables are exposed to and the time exposed to outside pathogens.

Convenience food industry—When I was young it was a rarity for a store to be open on Sunday. It truly was the day of rest. But no longer. An industry of "immediate calories" has developed over the last generation. Pizzas delivered to your home, delivery services bringing meals from a line-up of restaurants, microwavable calories, a network of convenience stores—all providing cheap, caloric-dense foods seven days a week. The idea of most U.S. citizens having such easy access to food is relativity new in human adaptation. Starvation and a constant search for food was the norm;calling a pizza delivery service is the exception. Just because these entities exist doesn't mean you have to patronize them. Other calorie cutting methods on this list will provide ideas on finding "satiety" (the feeling of fullness) and existing in a world with the convenience food industry without being a captive customer of their inexpensive, high-calorie offerings.

A personal tale related to the convenience food industry: My first job was working at a Texaco station. It was the era where we still came outside to pump customers' gas, check the oil and clean their windshields. The person who had the job before me quit. When I went to work, the owner didn't want to change the name on the uniform. During my gas station career, I was known as "Ron" to the customers. Cut forward to now. There may be a handful of stations left where an attendant pumps gas. The places where we refuel our vehicles now are multi-purpose facilities where we get gasoline but can also order breakfast, lunch, pizza, and select from a wide selection of baked goods, drinks (alcohol and non-) and candy. In the original version of "Cut Your Calories...Now!" (CYCN) it was suggested not to pay for gasoline inside the store. Pay outside at the pump with a debit card. Going into the store exposes one to a test of impulses where a Reese's Peanut Butter Cup with 210 calories can be purchased and consumed without giving it much thought. So, as a subset to Number 2, I'll repeat it: pay for your gasoline outside at the pump.

There is a convenience store I utilize. The food selection is so large and wide-ranging that they have a sit-down seating area inside. I was gassing up my Jeep one day when a message came on the screen. I just won a 22-ounce drink! All I had to do was buy a six-inch hoagie. I declined the offer and finished fueling up. When I tried to print the receipt, the message board told me the printer was broken and I had to get the receipt from the clerk. Was it set up that way? Were they going to do what was necessary to get me in the store? Probably not. But when I go into this particular store, I notice that the layout was done by somebody who knows how to bombard the hunger impulses of a person. Cookies are located right inside the front door. Food is on display everywhere in front of you. The walkway in the store leads you past impulse items. Straight ahead are both the cookie/candy aisles and the huge doughnut display case. Entering your peripheral vision to the immediate right is the menu board announcing all the items available from the kitchen. I do buy coffee there in the early a.m. I notice that when you turn from the coffee machines you are looking straight at the doughnut case. In my writing career, I have never once used the word "onslaught" but that's what this store is—an onslaught of food items. (One time I needed a phone charger for a trip. They had chargers but were in an area where you had to get off the "food path" to find them.)

Two final notes: I'm amazed at the stores that now sell impulse items. Best Buy, Office Depot, Michael's Crafts, and others. Why does the place where I get office supplies need to sell me Twizzlers and Snickers bars? And that Texaco station where I used to work? It's now a KFC, the fast food restaurant formerly known as Kentucky Fried Chicken.

Number 3 Don't Eat in Your Car

It's unhealthy, it's dangerous and you're paying attention to the road and not the calories you're consuming—a perfect recipe for overconsumption. Eating in your car also lowers the resale value of the vehicle.

Number 4 Appreciate the Power of the Restaurant Industry

The lower prices of foodstuff and the flow of capital to the restaurant industry have resulted in an explosion in restaurants and publicly-owned restaurant chains. The result: today there are three times the number of restaurants that there were 40 years ago. Fast food sites grew by 85% during the ten-year period ending in 1996. While the typical American is eating fewer than 1/3 of his or her meals away from home, more than 1/3 of total calories are consumed outside the house.

When I was growing up, my family was a "non-restaurant" family. We didn't have the means or the reason to go. But as I got into the business world and started traveling, I found myself in restaurants on a regular basis (in fact, too much!) One of the industries I'm active in runs on food. There is no shortage of industry members offering to buy me a meal, sponsor a food-oriented seminar, etc. I've overeaten in some of the finest establishments in some of the largest cities in the world. When I was engaged, my ex-fiancée (all 5'10" & 135 lbs. of her) was a full-time employee in the medical field and a student. I fell into the trap of taking her to dinner on a regular basis. She never gained an ounce but I, in spite of my swimming and bike riding, got to the point where I was wearing my overconsumption of calories. It became too easy to go to any one of the 25 chain restaurants located within a few miles of her house. Even with the knowledge of nutrition I had at that time, I left that knowledge in the car while I went inside to Olive Garden, TGI Friday's, P.F. Chang's, Red Robin, Red Lobster, Bob Evans, Mitchell's Seafood, Cheesecake Factory, Golden Corral, Longhorn Steakhouse...and on and on and on.

You have to learn the most effective and efficient manner to live in a society with such a large restaurant presence. Here are suggestions to navigate your restaurant visits:

1. Go in prepared to have one-half of your meal going home with you in a "to go" box.
2. Share servings with your dining partner(s).
3. Don't order appetizers except for times when you can create a meal from appetizers.
4. Don't eat the highly refined bread before dinner. The highly refined flour in the bread, eaten before a meal, may have immediate impact of lowering your blood sugar, creating a false sense of "hunger" and causing you to "over-order" and overeat.
5. Don't drink alcohol before ordering. Even one drink may cause your "impulse control" to go on vacation and you will over-order and overeat. I know many restaurant operators. I have firsthand experience of how restaurants operate. If I owned a restaurant and you had an 8:00 p.m. reservation and there was a table open, I would tell you there is a short wait. I would suggest you go to the bar and have a drink or two before dinner. I want you to check your coat and your impulse control before ordering.
6. You should "know" the menu of your favorite restaurants. If your meal plan for the day calls for a visit to a restaurant you frequent, include an offering you've had before in the

plan. This may reduce the risk of over ordering and overeating. I go to a local restaurant on a regular basis owned by a friend of mine. There are three items I select from. I don't even need to read the menu.

7. Go for fiber. If you're in a new spot, order a dish high in fiber. The fiber may come in the form of a salad, vegetables, beans or whole grains.

8. Use your restaurant visits as a place to eat fish. You can't go wrong with salmon or scallops but you may also want to try different fish and increase your Omega-3 fat consumption. I had my first dinner of trout earlier this year—in Johnstown, Pennsylvania of all places.

9. If you're a young man trying to woo a young lady and think the way to do it is to take her to dinner at an upscale restaurant, think again. What you really should be doing is learning how to cook, figuring out some interesting food combinations, investing in some quality cookware, and making a meal for the object of your affection.

Two final notes on restaurants: the food cost of a pizza establishment may be as low as 25% (compared with 33% for a typical full-service restaurant, expressed as a percentage of total sales). The number of independent and corporate-owned pizza establishments has probably grown faster than the overall restaurant rate of three times over 40 years. The founders of large franchise chains are celebrated as smart business people who have achieved great success. It's become common place for a family to eat pizza a few times per week. For young people, it's the favorite "post-drinking" meal. But we have to rethink our addiction to pizza.

Extremely cheap calories. The refined wheat used in the crust is identified as sugar by your body. The overconsumption of cheese in America is directly related to the obesity issue. Some pizza chains now inject cheese into the crust. Due to the competitive nature of the industry, "more is more" is the rule among pizza shops. But this pizza is unfamiliar to the people who live in Italy. Pizza in Italy has a thin crust and the toppings are few. No topping is there to provide a competitive advantage against the shop owner down the street. Pizza in Italy is made by people trained to make pizza. Here, in the chains and franchises, the process and ingredients are "dumb downed" so any new hire can make the product.

You have to start reducing two things from your diet: pizza and cheese. When I was younger, I didn't realize that cheese didn't naturally come wrapped in single slices. Kraft Foods (now Kraft Heinz), due to technology and a large Research & Development budget, found a way to reduce a process that takes an extended period of time and minimize it to a few days. This is not a paragraph telling you to eliminate pizza but it should be reduced. As for cheese, continue to buy it in blocks and slice it when needed but you really should eliminate the cheese slices from your diet. That product is not really cheese. It's something else.

Also: from the original CYCN brochure: Never eat at a restaurant with the word "buffet" above the door. The economics of the buffet restaurant are of interest. Because they're using lower-end serving dishes and aren't overspending on interior build-out, they are able to offer an "all you can eat" deal at a reasonable price. One study I read stated that the average price charged by a buffet restaurant is $12.95 per person and the food cost per person is less than $6.00—an attractive margin for any restaurant.

Number 5 Pay Attention to Portion Control

A few years ago, I read a story about a woman who bought an older house. The house was built in the 1950s and still had some of the original features. When she started to put her plates in the kitchen cupboard, she discovered they didn't fit. The older house had cupboards only big enough for the plates used at that time. Due to competitive issues, the "growing" of America (pun intended) includes the plates and cups used in our homes.

Barbara J. Rolls is a name I've been familiar with for many years. She is a Professor of Nutritional Sciences at Penn State University—and so much more. Review her CV online to get an understanding of her accomplishments. She is known for the term "Volumetrics," which, in the most simplistic definition, means, "People will eat the food placed in front of them."

To practice portion control, here are four suggestions:

- Like the woman in the story mentioned above, buy smaller serving dishes *(I assume she did that instead of buying larger cabinets)*.
- Make vegetables a larger portion of the meal, not by adding additional vegetables but by substituting them for a part of the higher calorie animal protein.
- Do not bring the serving dish, crockpot or platter to the dining room table. Leave it in the kitchen. This will reduce the risk of people at the table "grazing" after finishing their meal.

- If possible, don't serve yourself. If you're eating with others, have the family members/guests prepare the plates of others.

And this only has a slight correlation here but it is of interest: People tend to consume more calories based on an increased number of people at a table. Strange but true. It reminds me of the many times I went to a party, business meeting, wedding, etc., and had my impulse control lowered by alcohol and ended up consuming way too many calories. Part of it was the occasion, part of it was the alcohol, and part of it, I'm sure, was the size of the plates of my fellow diners.

Number 6 Limit Your Dinner Selection
Years ago, I read that the average family has a dinner selection chosen from 14 different items. When I think back to my household, that number appears about right. There was a rotation my mother used to feed her family. Instead of reaching for new dishes and recipes for the sake of something new, settle on a short list of meals you can prepare for dinner. Make the meals filling, easy to prepare, use the pre-cut peppers and onions (see Number 1), and structure the ingredients so that the overall meal remains low on the Glycemic Index.

Note: I constantly see great recipes online. And there are probably equally great recipes in the celebrity cookbooks and weight loss books that support a large percentage of the publishing industry. But there is a major disconnect going on here. Despite all these recipes and all these cookbooks, the American waistline continues to expand. You don't need to keep adding dishes to your dinner selection. You'll see this phrase again: less is more.

Time for a contradiction. I just wrote that you need to limit the number of meal options you and your family should have to select from for dinner. One man who may disagree with me is James A. Duke. Dr. Duke was trained in botany, developed the USDA's Phytochemical and Ethnobotanical database, and is known for trips to the Amazon rain forest in search of plants that can be converted into medicines. In his journeys, he would travel with local shaman into the forests to select the plants for study. The shaman knew which plants were used to treat ailments among the locals.

Dr. Duke, while famous for many things, is most famous to me for this quote about nutrition: "Moderation in everything...except variety."

Dr. Duke is telling you to try new foods, experiment, reach out, and explore new tastes and cuisine from other countries. And, in spite of what I just wrote, I agree with him. I wish I had access to the vegetable "Morning Glory" (pak boong) I would eat every day in Thailand. This vegetable looks much like asparagus but without the sharp aftertaste.

In Cuba, yuca (spelled with one "c") is served with almost every dinner. Yuca, also known as cassava, is a staple food in South and Latin America. It is complex carbohydrate-dense, low in fat, and high in fiber and potassium. It is prepared boiled, baked or grilled. I could eat yuca every day. I am always amazed at what the "food magicians" do in Cuba. As more private restaurants are opening, a visitor to the island should be having all their meals from the growing "sector privado" (private sector). On my last trip I was impressed with a simple cabbage salad (which I added to my culinary offerings) and what the private restaurants were doing with peppers to add flavor to the pork and chicken dinners (orange bell peppers were used constantly).

What I'm saying is this: if you find healthy fare from another country and you can incorporate it into your limited selection for dinner, do so. At this time, yuca is not readily available where I live. If it becomes so, I will certainly be a buyer.

Last note on James Duke: when he was in college, he played in a jazz band. He came to my hometown a number of years ago and gave a speech about his work. At the end, he brought out a ukulele and accompanied himself while he sang a song about botanicals, their nicknames, and their various uses.

Number 7 Become a Vegetarian 2 to 3 Days Each Week; Become Wheat-Free 2 to 3 Days Per Week

I'm not a vegetarian. I eat eggs almost daily in omelets and I eat pork chops and fish on a regular basis. But I aspire to be a vegetarian. Not for religious reasons and not because I'm consuming something that was once alive. The documentaries *Fast Food Nation, Food, Inc.*, and the classic novel, *The Jungle* by Upton Sinclair have to give us all second thoughts about consuming animal protein.

I aspire to be a vegetarian for low-calorie and economic reasons. Animal protein is always more expensive than plant-based protein. I pick two or three days per week when I am a vegetarian. No meat, no dairy. I still eat eggs in my breakfast omelet but load up on beans, vegetables, penne pasta, barley, and the cut-up peppers I prepared for the week (a related note: Dr. Andrew Weil, known for his involvement in Integrative Medicine, once listed the glycemic index of various forms of pasta. He wrote that penne is the lowest (slowest to convert to glucose) on the index;it has to deal with the way the penne is formed.) On my "veggie" days I sometimes eat sleek and fattoush from a local restaurant owned by a Lebanese family. If you don't know what those two dishes are, I'm suggesting strongly that you find a spot that serves them and eat "outside the box."

Inversely, if we're going to be occasional vegetarians (not "vegans" who do not consume any eggs, fish, or dairy), we should also be "wheat-free" 2 to 3 days per week. Are you familiar with a book titled *Wheat Belly*? If not, you should become acquainted. I've read at least 125 nutrition and health-related books and I have to rank *Wheat Belly* in the Top Ten. The book was written by William Davis, M.D., a cardiologist from Wisconsin. The book was published in 2011 and, like other best-selling nutrition books, has spawned related books. Dr. Davis' theories of wheat consumption leading to obesity/Type II diabetes/food addiction are disagreed upon by others in the NAI (Nutrition Advice Industry). Any best-selling nutrition book that is opposite of the NAI's accepted guidelines is challenged. However, I found his book to be insightful and presented well. I've known for a long time that when you can almost totally refine a carbohydrate (as in wheat to flour) your body will identify the fiber-lacking product as sugar.

Here is my take on William Davis's book, and it starts with the achievements of a great man, Norman Borlaug. Borlaug was a trained biologist who helped various countries to become more effective and efficient in developing their farmland and increasing wheat production. His quote was (paraphrased), "A country has to feed its population." Borlaug worked with Mexico to make their wheat production high-yielding and disease resistant. More production was done on less land. While Borlaug didn't introduce GMO (Genetically Modified Organisms) to the crop, he did change the "amber waves of grain" (which were and are subject to weather destruction) to semi-dwarf/multiline status which was more resistant to disease.

Borlaug later introduced his methods to Pakistan,

India, and various Asian/African countries. For his efforts, he received the Nobel Peace Prize in 1970, the Presidential Medal of Freedom, and the Congressional Gold Medal (one of only seven people to achieve this Triple Crown). Borlaug also received India's second high civilian prize, the Padma Vibhushan.

Norman Borlaug did a great thing. What William Davis states is that the cross-breeding efforts changed the chemical composition of wheat. Wheat is now a highly refined, fiber-free grain with addictive qualities, and extremely high on the glycemic index. Davis points out in his book that the glycemic index of white bread is higher than that of table sugar. And because this flour is so cheap, it's used in so many different products. Next time you're in a supermarket, check out the bread aisle—which has tripled over the last generation (my estimate)—the cereal aisle (same thing), and the cookie/cracker aisle. All foods with a base of highly refined wheat. We are eating too much highly refined wheat. Dr. Davis suggests we be 100% wheat-free. I'm suggesting a start by eliminating flour-based products 2-3 days per week.

Number 8 Measure Your Pasta

While we just discussed *Wheat Belly* and Dr. Davis's claims that you should be wheat-free, it is difficult to live that lifestyle. I've read the book and recommend it highly, but, while I've reduced my wheat product consumption, I'm not wheat-free. Not everybody will be able to live wheat-free. Let's start with a simple step: Pay attention to the amount of pasta you are eating per serving. When I used to make angel hair, linguine, or penne pasta, I had no idea how much I was eating. I just eyeballed the dry pasta and threw it in the boiling water. My first step in learning the process of measuring pasta was when a chef on the radio said that one serving of spaghetti covered the area of a quarter when placed on end. So I did that for a while. Then I found a serving spoon with holes cut out in the handle that measured various sizes of spaghetti per serving. I used that for a while. Then I talked to the owner of an Italian eatery. He told me that one serving of noodle pasta equals four ounces. One serving of penne equals one cup. By following this advice, you won't over-prepare pasta (I've thrown out a lot over the years) and you won't overeat the finished product.

Number 9 Don't Eat Anything Where the Marketing Cost Per Unit is Greater Than the Total Cost of the Ingredients Per Unit

A long title, I know. But one that is near and dear to me. William Blake, the great English novelist and poet (and a major influence on Jim Morrison) once wrote, "To generalize is to be an idiot." At the risk of sounding like an idiot, I am going to generalize

Think of a food product where the packaging and advertising cost per unit is greater than the sum total of the ingredients. What could that be? That's right: cereal. Like you, I ate a ton of it as a kid. I dug my hand into the bottom of full boxes in search of that elusive prize, I read the back of the box while digesting the contents and once I even asked my father if putting chocolate milk on Rice Krispies would result in Cocoa Krispies (it didn't). I also ate cereal as an adult. I consumed countless bowls of Shredded Wheat or the generic version of Cheerios with rice milk.

But no more. I no longer drink milk—rice, soy, or almond. Those products aren't milk, they're flavored water drinks. As for cow's milk, the evidence is in favor of not drinking it. It is the only animal product with sugar, has zero phytonutrients ("phyto" is the

Greek word for plant), and zero fiber. Ask yourself this question: what species continues to drink milk after it's weaned from its mother? Humans. That's all. In spite of what the Milk Marketing Board tells you, milk does not do a body good. If you're going to talk about the need for calcium, especially among growing children and older adults, I'm going to refer you to this important study: "Worldwide incidence of hip fracture in elderly women: relation to consumption of animal and vegetable foods." (*European Journal of Nutrition* 2001; 40: 200-13) The study analyzed hip fracture incidence (HFI) among women 50 years old plus in 33 countries.

The study concluded that the **"...critical determinant of hip fracture risk in relation to the acid-base effects of diet is the net load of acid in the diet, when the intake of both acid and base precursors is considered. Moderation of animal food consumption and an increased ratio of vegetable/animal food consumption may confer a protective effect."** In addition, early on in my nutrition studies I read reports stating that cultures with the lowest rate of dairy product consumption have the lowest rates of osteoporosis (i.e. Asian countries). In summary, at least one major study and epidemiology states that high dairy product consumption doesn't prevent osteoporosis but causes it.

Back to the cereal bowl. Many of us were helped along with our "sugar love" with the high-sugar cereals we ate as children. To this day, I remember how good it tasted to drink the milk from the bottom of the bowl. Why was it good? Because some of the sugar came off the cereal and found its way into the milk. The "sugar milk" was delicious.

If you want to defend your cereal choice as one high in fiber, you may need to change your defense. Some of the high-fiber cereals have a base of refined grains with fiber added back (sometimes in the form of miller's bran).

I know it's easy to grab the cereal box. I know most children are happy eating sugar-carrying cereal but it is a source of empty calories. As consumers and as parents, we have to find other ways to begin our nutrition day instead of eating high-profit margin, (oftentimes) high-sugar cereal made from highly refined grains. Some of those ways are provided throughout this list.

There are other food products where the marketing cost is greater than the product cost. Off hand, I would list many snack foods, sodas, highly processed and packaged foods, and foods that are highly advertised on TV. Before buying or eating a food, give some thought to the marketing effort used to get you to buy it and eat it.

On that note, in a book that became a nutrition classic as soon as it was published, *Salt Sugar Fat,* by Michael Moss (published in 2013 with the subtitle of *How the Food Giants Hooked Us*), Moss shares the story of a cereal company that hired an advertising executive to run the business. The company knew their product was the same as the other dozens of cereal companies. They needed a creative guy to beat the others where it counted most—on the TV ads, especially the ones aimed at children.

Number 10 "Paper vs. Plastic"

Purchase your food with paper money and not debit or credit cards. The folding money has more value to you than do credit cards. I don't care if you have to walk to the ATM to get cash before visiting your favorite restaurant or going food shopping, having cash to spend means you'll spend less. Who says so? McDonald's. They issued a report stating that the average credit card user spent $7.00 per purchase vs. $4.50 for the average cash buyer. And Dun & Bradstreet, the credit profiling company, reports that consumers spend 12% to 18% more on purchases (food and non-food) when using credit cards instead of cash.

Cash has more value than credit cards to you even though the purchasing power is equal. Debit cards are in the middle of these two forms of payment and the same principal applies. You overspend on food when using any type of plastic.

Number 11 Replace Your Gatorade with Electrolyte Tablets

As I write this, there is a bottle of Gatorade Fierce on my desk. The flavor is irrelevant. The bottle contains 28 ounces. The label says this is equivalent to 2.5 servings. If I were on a bike ride or running bleacher steps, I would drink the entire bottle in no time at all and be looking for more. The label says the amount of sugar per serving is 21 grams. When I started my journey on the nutrition learning curve, I was taught that the amount of sugar that fits on a teaspoon was 4.72 grams. An internet search now states it as 4 grams per teaspoon. For rounding purposes, we'll use the lower figure. There are 5.25 teaspoons of sugar per serving. I would (and I have) consumed 13.125 teaspoons full of sugar in a few minutes. The 28-ounce bottle, where 2.5 servings is one serving in reality, would cause me to consume a total of 200 calories.

Gatorade is owned by PepsiCo. Their logo is in every sports arena, on every sideline, and their name is ubiquitous with sports drinks. This company spends tens of millions of dollars per year for naming rights, licensing fees and other advertising channels for a product that is 93% water and a lot of sugar.

I think PepsiCo realized that the growing backlash against heavy sugar drinks would affect them so they invested in Propel, a zero-calorie, flavored drink. (PepsiCo and Coke both saw the handwriting on the wall years ago and purchased bottled water companies.) I used Propel for many years until I saw the light. I now use electrolyte tablets. I drop two of them in a gallon container of water, shake up the container, and fill my water bottle from the container. End result: I'm getting electrolytes with a small percentage of the calories Gatorade has, I'm spending far less money on sports drinks, and I'm not responsible for so many empty plastic bottles ending up in the landfill. I get my electrolyte tablets at a camping/hiking store but have also seen them in bicycle shops. *I once gave a glass of the Lemon + Lime electrolyte water to a visitor. They remarked that it tasted "...just like Mountain Dew but without the sugar!"*

Number 12 Teach Your Children the Economics of Food

It's never too early to start. Most of us probably developed our refined carbohydrate and sugar reliance (saving the word "addiction") before we were old enough to realize what messages the advertising industry was sending us. I'm a believer in education and reinforcement of that education. My step-daughter was about 11 years old and needed to pack a lunch for a school event. In the store, the colorful box of a Lunchables container jumped out at her. She didn't know the history of this product, the fact that a cigarette maven applied the techniques of nicotine marketing to help make Lunchables a $1 billion-per-year product and she didn't understand the profit margin that Oscar Mayer (and its parent Kraft Heinz) would make from us. She hadn't bothered to read the label for nutritional content and she certainly didn't know that highly compensated graphic artists, brilliant in appealing to the 11-year-old brain, designed that package to prevent her from looking elsewhere. Lastly, she didn't give any thought to the fact that the supermarket was probably paid a handsome fee to have the Lunchables placed right where they were.

I did my best to explain to her that there were a lot of smart people who knew how to market to her. At this stage in her life, it was going to be through me, her mother, and her grandparents. But growing up, she would receive an endless stream of messages from sellers of products, food and otherwise, who were trying to separate her from her money. Sometimes the seller would give less to her in value than the value she surrendered. She was able to comprehend what I was sharing with her and read for herself the fat and sodium content of this manufactured food. She was also able to understand that we had limited resources to spend on food and that we needed to make better food choices. She went a step further and started reading food labels on a regular basis and even studied the "cost per ounce" labels on the supermarket shelf.

As I write this, I remember thinking how easy it was to share this insight with her. I don't know that I would have responded in the same way if one of my parents tried to educate me on why my interest in Sugar Frosted Flakes wasn't a wise one.

Number 13 Don't Use the Supplement Industry or Pharmaceutical Industry as an Excuse to Overconsume

Remember "Fen-Phen?" The combination of prescription weight loss drugs Phentermine and Fenfluramine was a big seller in 1996. The industry was sure this was the pharmaceutical industry's answer to the growing obesity issue. You couldn't turn on a talk show or pick up a newspaper without hearing about or reading about the magic of Fen-Phen. Millions of prescriptions were sold in that first year.

In 1997, Fen-Phen was banned because it critically damaged users' heart valves. The pharma industry will never give up in a search for an FDA-approved weight loss drug that they can sell through the medical profession. If you're a fan of marketing, think of all the free advertising an approved weight loss drug will receive. After a 13-year break, the Food and Drug Administration (FDA) approved two weight-loss drugs in 2012. There is a theory that, with the increased costs of obesity and the Affordable Care Act's (ACA) focus on prevention, that the FDA may approve more drugs in the pipeline with somewhat less favorable results in trials than pre-ACA.

So here is the question: Do you think anybody who was prescribed Fen-Phen took their daily dosage after eating a large pizza? After returning home from the buffet restaurant? It's a rhetorical question, so no answer is needed.

In my darkest days, I worked in the body building-supplement business. I've got enough stories from those dark days to write an illuminating book. I've always kept my eyes and ears open to that industry. Another question: Do you think anybody got so excited about the new "fat burning" pill being sold at the local supplement store that they celebrated by having dinner at their favorite fast food restaurant? Again, no answer required.

Do not use any product pushed by the pharma/supplement industries to rationalize overconsumption of calories.

And this is the perfect time for a great story. When I first started doing seminars, I was presenting at a large law firm in downtown Pittsburgh. The venue was in the firm's auditorium. They brought half of the workforce in and I did a seminar. The second half came in, and I did another seminar.

Some of the employees were hearing-impaired so there were two interpreters converting what I was saying into sign language.

During the first seminar, a woman asked if she should use supplements. I told her this: If she ate too much food, not enough essential fat, not enough fiber, too much sugar, if she smoked, abused alcohol, if she didn't have enough physical activity and didn't get enough sleep, that there would not be a pill, powder, mixer or elixir that would do her one bit of good. Nobody can disagree with what I told that woman *unless they're in the supplement business.*

As that seminar was ending, another woman approached me. She told me she had the perfect idea on how to use supplements. I told her I was always looking to learn and wanted to hear what she had to say. She proceeded to tell me that the only time she used supplements was "...on the days that I eat at fast food restaurants." I have told that story many times, to small groups and in one-on-one settings. Most people laugh out loud at the silly rationalization. But there are others who look at me and nod as if they think the woman was on to something. But guess what? She wasn't.

PART TWO: THE PHYSICAL ASPECTS OF CALORIE CUTTING

Number 14 H.A.L.T.S. (plus a few)

A common acronym in nutrition education, H.A.L.T.S. stands for the following:

H   Hunger
OK, so you think you're hungry. Your stomach (or most likely your brain) has announced that you're hungry. Let's run through the checklist.

A   Anger
Are you angry at something or someone? Chances are you may want to take out your anger on food. Not the cause? Continue.

L   Lazy
Maybe you're just having a lazy day/week/life. Your brain is not thinking of anything related to your life/work/creative pursuits. When that happens, your brain will think of food. If this is the cause of your hunger, and you know you will be eating a meal in the next few hours, maybe you can do something productive or physical to change your brain's craving.

T   Tired
Important factor. Our brains are wired to constantly crave easy-to-digest carbohydrates. I've experienced the horrible sensation of needing to eat to generate energy to stay

awake and get important work done. There are multiple reasons for this type of fatigue. One of them could be dehydration. Even if you're not physically thirsty, you may benefit from increasing your water intake. If this is why you're hungry, have some water, do some exercise, or switch to a different work project that may result in increased enthusiasm.

S   Stress
I know few people who would say stress doesn't make them want to eat. The genesis to this mechanism may be found in our ancestors, whose stress could have been caused by certain dangers that no longer exist in our world. They may have felt a stressful situation was going to result in a questionable food supply for an unknown period and they needed to eat in order to store calories for a period of unknown food supply. It may be that chewing desirable food creates endorphins that, momentarily, get our minds off the stressful situation (similar to cigarette smoking and the creation of dopamine). There are ways to minimize certain stress factors and eliminate others, shared elsewhere in this document.

Here are two more "brain triggers" that may cause us to overeat:

R&B   Restless & Bored (also a cool type of music!)
This one applies to many of us but to me in droves. I was a hyperactive kid and I became a hyperactive adult. If I can't be doing something productive and creative, I have no issue being productive and creative with

food. I appreciate my hyperactive nature because it provided me with the energy to get an education I didn't deserve, develop interests I otherwise wouldn't have, travel, write, develop an entrepreneurial nature, and to be involved in sports and other physical pursuits the vast majority of my life. But when my "creative soul" (credit to Bruce Springsteen for that term) is not being fed, I can easily convince myself I'm hungry when I'm probably really not. The cure? The same as listed under "T." On a personal level, you know the projects you're involved with. You can divert your hunger to one of these projects or do something else to turn your mind away from the thought of food. Most often, it is your brain telling you you're hungry and not your physical body.

M   Memory
There are times when the idea of eating something pops into my head. I have eaten things because the thought came in, food was close by and I had the ability to get it. But no more. Now when I think of eating, I check with my memory. My sudden hunger doesn't remember that I ate two hours ago and I'll be eating again in the near future. My brain is overriding my memory. When this happens, I have to check with my memory to see how recently I ate and how close I am to my next meal or snack.

Number 15 "Hara Hachi Bu"

This is a Japanese term that roughly translates to "Eat until you are eight parts full" or "belly 80 percent full." It has gotten the most attention among people on the island of Okinawa which has the world's highest percentage of population over 100 years of age. (Okinawan females have the longest life span and life expectancy among any country's female population.) Not only is "Hara Hachi Bu" part of the reason for the long life expectancy due to its reduced calorie consumption—which results in a lower Body Mass Index—but Okinawans live a Spartan-type existence. They have minimal furniture and eat their meals sitting cross-legged on the floor. Part of their longevity is attributed to the fact that they have to get down to floor level and back up a few times per day. How many 70-year-olds do you know who can easily sit on the floor and get back up?

This concept has a physiologic base in a hormone called "leptin." Leptin is the "satiety hormone" which is produced in the adipose cells in your midsection. The hormone travels to your brain and tells the hippocampus that you are full and can stop eating. The problem is that the journey is not immediate. It may take 20 minutes or so for the message to be delivered. It is in this 20-minute period that we can do a lot of damage with a knife and fork. I think this concept fits perfectly with Barbara Rolls' work on portion control. If you start out with a plate 80% full, you may not need to worry about the leptin delivery messenger service working perfectly. One of the theories about obesity is that a percentage of the population has zero leptin receptors in their brain and overeats because their brain is not delivering a "Full—stop eating!" message. One of the problems with alcohol consumption (my theory only) is that the alcohol drowns out the leptin message and causes one to overeat.

Lastly, I don't think we do a good job of "eyeballing" our plates. I have walked out of many restaurants and have left the dinner table at many holiday meals with that feeling of being bloated. That's an awful feeling. I ate way too much. I didn't use portion control and I probably had enough alcohol pre-meal to dull my leptin mechanism. But I should have taken a good look at the food on my plate and determined which percentage of it was coming home with me. I ate way too much many times but not anymore. I now have the tools to prevent that horrible bloated feeling.

Number 16 Drink Water Before Meals

There is an oft-cited study from the journal *Obesity*. The study divided 48 adults between the ages of 55 and 75 into two groups. Each group was put on a low-calorie (compared to today's standards) diet of 1,200 calories (for women) and 1,500 calories for men. One-half of the participants were told to drink water before each of three daily meals. Three months later, the "water" group had lost about 15 pounds each while the "dry" group lost about 11 pounds each. Each group was going to lose weight because they probably each lowered the daily amount of calories they were consuming. The footnote to the study is that the groups were reviewed 12 months later. The "water" group had kept up with the habit of drinking H2O before meals and lost an additional 1.5 pounds, whereas the other group had regained their weight.

This study is all over the internet. One has to wonder why two groups eating the same calories per day lost different amounts of weight. Why would water make the difference? It could be that the water consumed before the meal caused the glucose/insulin response to happen more slowly and may have led that group to not "cheat" between meals. Or they may even have consumed less than the allotted calories at each subsequent meal.

Here's my take on water before meals:

1. The water may steer you away from sugar-free sodas, which may cause some disruption with the digestive process.
2. One of the causes of fatigue is dehydration. Many fatigued people graze on cheap carbohydrates in order to get energy to conduct their daily chores. Regular consumers of water may be less fatigued and be prone to less grazing (and have more physical activity in their lives).
3. The water may even take the place of alcohol calories and prevent a loss of impulse control. You don't need special bottled water to increase your water consumption. Most of the water in those bottles comes from the public water supply.
4. Get a nice charcoal filter for your tap or even use the electrolyte tablets described in Number 11. Less plastic in the landfill.

One of my clients runs a large business. He has many demands on his time. I met him in the gym we trained in years ago. He was effective and efficient with his workout time. Others were there to do the same thing day after day and socialize and then wonder why their results were minimal. Not this guy. He knew what he was doing. He starts his day by drinking two larges glasses of water and doing some yoga stretches. He probably weighs the same amount or less than he did 20 years ago. Good genetics? Knowledge about nutrition? Effective and efficient workouts? Water before breakfast? Probably "yes" to all four but he's a testament to pre-meal water.

Number 17 Say Good-bye to Fruit Juice

I can almost hear the Nutrition Advice Industry ranting about this one but let me make a case. The healthy part of a fruit is in the fiber and the phytonutrients that are stripped away to deliver the end result: fruit-flavored sugar water. In an 8-ounce glass of orange juice, there are 22 grams of sugar. Using our 4-gram per tablespoon, that 8-ounce glass just gave us 5.5 teaspoons of sugar. And I think the Referenced Amount Customarily Consumed (RACC) on the label is misleading. Most of us would consume more than 8 ounces.

The "calorie consumption" connection is that a glass of orange juice at breakfast may cause a spike in glucose levels and the accompanying insulin response, which will lower your blood sugar to a level lower than it was "pre-juice." This may cause an overconsumption of breakfast calories.

The orange industry did a great job of marketing themselves. Few people in my age range don't know the expression, "Breakfast without orange juice is like a day without sunshine," and the ex-spokesperson for the Florida Citrus Commission, Anita Bryant. Ms. Bryant was a singer with some success who began to tout orange juice in 1969 through constant TV commercials. Growing up, orange juice was always in the refrigerator. The marketing blitz worked. But Ms. Bryant couldn't help but let her anti-gay sentiments get in the way of a good paycheck. She was vocal in her negative feelings about gays. There was a time when gay bars stopped serving screwdrivers, which required orange juice, and replaced them with "Anita Bryants," made with vodka and apple juice. A Who's Who of celebrities of that era got involved with the boycott of Florida oranges. Ms. Bryant's contract was allowed to run out in 1979 and she faded into Wikipedia fame.

Don't drink fruit juice. Parents give children fruit juice thinking the fruit component has value. But it really doesn't. It's just helping to develop a reliance on sugar. A better call is water. Get children away from soda and juices when they're young. Introduce them to water.

On two personal notes, the only time I drink orange juice now is during my once-per-year sinus infection; a remnant from a broken nose playing football in tenth grade. And to this day, when I eat an orange, I eat the inside of the peel when I'm done with the fruit. That is a habit developed when I was on the wrestling team. When your match was over, and you were leaving the mat, Coach Harding would toss an orange to you. He always brought a shopping bag full of oranges. We had nowhere to throw the peels so we started eating the insides.

Pop quiz!! What is the white inside part of an orange called? Hint: it contains four letters and the first letter is "p" but it is not "pulp." What is it?

In closing this section, I think there is one other food group that has used extensive marketing efforts, government assistance, and capital investment in a successful effort to convince the American population that their product is healthy like orange juice. It is a fan favorite of the Nutrition Advice Industry but not me. I'm not a fan of this food. I do, however, respect the marketing job producers of this food have done. If we meet, ask me what it is.

Number 18 Oatmeal—Not Just for Breakfast Anymore!!

I have been an oatmeal junkie for a long time. One of my "oatmeal memories" was having a bowl of oatmeal compote in the coffee shop of the Beverly Hills Hotel. "Compote" is a French word meaning fruit cooked in syrup. My memory is that the oatmeal had bits of red and green apples, raisins and brown sugar. My other memory is that one bowl of oatmeal cost $14.95.

I have had many bowls of the microwaveable oatmeal with a banana and vanilla yogurt. I knew the yogurt was high in sugar and had zero fiber but the taste combination was delicious. When I returned to the nutrition trade, I went another direction—then I reversed that direction.

When I originally wrote this section, I raved about the benefits of steel cut oats. Steel cut oats are a less refined version of what I had been eating for years. They can't be microwaved. On the stove, they take about 30 minutes to prepare. They have to be stirred on a regular basis. A great invention would be a spoon that would sit on the edge of a pot and stir itself every few minutes. A timer could be set to adjust how often the contents of the pot would be stirred. A person could be getting themselves or their family ready for work or school while the steel cut oats were cooking. A popular phrase for changing your direction is "walking back." I am walking back my devotion to steel cut oats. I ate them for a long period of time and (my opinion) they didn't keep my satiated (or "full") any longer than the regular microwaveable oatmeal I had been using. Steel cut oats may have a different impact on your personal level of fullness. What you put in the oatmeal may also result in the Glycemic Index being higher or lower. My suggestion here is to eat more oatmeal. Experiment with steel cut oats and different toppings—banana and yogurt, banana and brown sugar, crushed pineapple, raisins, etc. You can also find a few compote recipes you like and add them to the rotation.

Steel cut oats are used to make that children's story favorite—porridge. In the United Kingdom, steel cut oats are known as pinhead oatmeal or Scottish oats. I have a photo of myself eating porridge in Edinburgh, Scotland.

Number 19 **Go Out of Your Way to Get Fiber (or Fibre) into Your Diet**

When I started reading nutrition books and periodicals and interviewing dieticians, I often read, or was told, that we should strive to consume 35 grams of fiber per day but that the typical American was only eating about 10 grams of daily fiber. That was a long time ago. I could go online today and find countless articles stating we should be consuming 35 grams of fiber per day but, on average, we're only consuming 10 grams.

The message has been consistent but the results haven't changed. People don't eat enough fiber. Why not?

My theories:

- The profit margin on fiber-rich foods is lower than the profit margin on refined/processed/packaged foods. The fiber-poor foods are promoted more and get better shelf space in the stores. The processed/packaged/refined food industry is based on flour and not fibrous foods.
- We are still an animal protein-consuming nation. There is not one iota of fiber in any animal product so a daily animal protein consumer is going to have to go out of their way to include fiber in their diet.
- Fiber-low individuals may not have been exposed to the different types of beans they can use and the many food combinations they can make from beans.

The reasons for increasing fiber consumption include better control of blood sugar, a feeling of satiety, and decreased "transit time" (which has nothing to do with how long it takes you to get to work). Since fiber is classified as a carbohydrate and contains 4 calories per gram, there is another benefit directly related to this list. Fiber is consumed but not absorbed. By consuming 30 grams per day, it is the equivalent of reducing your calorie intake by 120 calories. The physiological reaction is probably not that direct but I've been carrying around a summary of a study done by the USDA stating that an increase in fiber consumption results in a decrease in calorie consumption.

Here are ways to incorporate more fiber into your diet:

Eat more oatmeal and incorporate steel cut oats into your diet (see Number 18). Introduce—or reintroduce—yourself to grits.

Get introduced to different beans/vegetable combinations. Before returning to the "nutrition trade," I used a lot of kidney beans. I now eat black beans, garbanzo beans, black-eyed peas, white beans, and pinto beans on a regular basis. It was only recently that I learned that pinto beans are used to make the refried beans so common in Mexican restaurants. I started doing "colander cooking," which is not cooking at all. I throw in white beans or black-eyed peas or chickpeas (a.k.a garbanzo beans) in the steel colander, throw in tuna, black olives, and onions, and have a meal. The same colander is used for three-bean salads. Low-cost, low preparation time, high in fiber, fulfilling meals. A creative cook at a diner I frequent uses beans in his omelets. This makes for a healthy and filling breakfast.

There are many reasons to eat beans. A short list:

1. Dynamite source of soluble fiber
2. Low on the Glycemic Index
3. High in vitamins and minerals
4. A natural protein-carbohydrate combination
5. Inexpensive (compared to animal protein)

And, maybe the most important member of the list:

6. "Beans are good sources of fuel for the health-promoting bacteria that live in your gut. We each have about two to four pounds of gut bacteria that strongly influence our immune system. In fact, about 70 percent of our immune response is generated from the gut. The bacteria love to eat the undigested raffinose, a type of carbohydrate, provided by beans and other vegetables such as broccoli, cauliflower, cabbage, Brussels sprouts and asparagus. Having well-nourished gut microbes invests in overall good health. A strong intake of prebiotics or bacteria food helps strengthen the immune system and optimizes wellness. In contracts, antibiotics kill the good bacteria along with the bad bacteria."

The above was excerpted from Nancy Clark, MS, RD, CSSD (specialist in sports dietetics). Ms. Clark's *Sports Nutrition Guidebook* is now in its 5th edition. I read the first edition (published in 1990) many years ago and still have copies of pages I made on a copying machine.

In case you missed what Ms. Clark was saying, the reason why people have gas is not because they've eaten beans but because they're *not eating enough of them.* I don't know that I agree with Ms. Clark. It may be that certain people have certain gut bacteria that diffuses the raffinose created by certain bean types. It may also happen that some people start to increase their consumption of beans but are turned away from an increase in gas. These people may not have given their intestines time enough to adjust to the increased raffinose. In any event, I don't think gas/flatulence is a reason not to utilize a nutritional powerhouse that has been proven to reduce calories, in both studies and in epidemiology. As long as there has been a human race, there has been flatulence. On an ironic note, an increase in bean-protein meals and a corresponding decline in animal protein would result in fewer beef cattle. Cattle are major producers of greenhouse gasses due to their flatulence. So, if you connect the dots: More beans = less global warming.

In the same way an increase in beans could result in fewer calories, cruciferous vegetables should be increased as a way to cut calories and promote better health. Cruciferous vegetables get their name from the cross-bearing shape of their flowers whose four petals resemble a cross.

You know the members of this family: broccoli, cauliflower, cabbage, Brussels sprouts, kale, bok choy, etc. The fiber per serving is between 3 and 6 grams and all members of this family are high in phytonutrients.

You can incorporate more of these vegetables in omelets, in penne pasta, and you can add broccoli or cabbage to your Sunday afternoon "prep time" when you're cutting up peppers, onions, tomatoes, etc. for use during the week. The same creative cook I mentioned above uses arugula in his breakfast specials. A tasty way to introduce an unsung, but valuable food, to his customers. One of the cruciferous members I've begun using since coming back to the trade is red cabbage. One of the most versatile, satisfying foodstuffs available. Don't look for the television commercial, though. Like the other food sources that are healthy, the low profit margin of these foods results in no advertising agency coming up with creative ads.

In studying the value of fiber, one will come across "resistant starches" (RS). RS are so named because the amylose polysaccharides are resistant to the digestion process. RS are sometimes referred to as the third type of dietary fiber, after insoluble and soluble. RS act similarly in the digestion process as fiber but are not distinguished on food labels. RS are found in many of the same foods as fiber and are classified as RS1 – RS4. RS4 is the "industry" resistant starch that is added back into breads and cereals. It does not occur naturally but is processed from corn. I've given up on bread as a fiber source due to the base of refined flour. And since I no longer eat cereal, I'm not worried about increasing my fiber/resistant starch from fortified cereals. But for a large percentage of the non-fiber eating population, foods containing RS or fortified with RS4 provide a way to obtain the healthy benefits of low glycemic index foods.

Two notes: I used the spelling "fibre" in introducing this section. That was a tribute to one of the most important nutrition books ever written. The book is *The Saccharine Disease* written by a British surgeon T.L. (Thomas Latimer) Cleave. Dr. Cleave was known for researching and writing about the negative effects of consuming refined carbohydrates. The ability to almost fully refine a carbohydrate is a relatively modern development. Cleave, to me, is most noted for "The Rule of 20," which states that 20 years after a society achieves the ability to refine carbohydrates, that society will experience a marked increase in Type II diabetes. Cleave's classic book, published in 1975, was a major influence on Dr. Robert Atkins and was a genesis for his work in developing the Atkins Diet and related books. I have a copy of this book borrowed from a library. I realized its significance and was worried I wouldn't see it again. I told the library I lost it, paid the fine, and am glad I did. This is one of the most important, yet least known, nutrition books. Most members of the Nutrition Advice Industry have never heard of Dr. Cleave or the Rule of 20 and, based on my personal experience, have no interest in learning about Cleave's work. In the book, Cleave uses the English spelling "fibre" instead of the Americanized "fiber."

While preparing this section, I ate an avocado. Not mixed with anything. Over the last year I have learned how to pick avocados, how to store them, how to open them, and what foods to prepare them with. On occasion, I scoop one out, put a little salt on the "meat" and eat it plain. The internet tells me that one California avocado has about 6 grams of fiber (maybe this is one thing on the internet we can believe). An avocado also contains a large amount of the important nutrient that will be discussed in Number 20.

Number 20 Fat is Your Friend!

Many years ago, when I was starting on the nutrition learning curve, I was in a club. Two girls were sitting at the bar. They were both well dressed. The girl on the right was thin. Her friend was a bigger girl. I approached the girl on the right. I included the bigger girl in the conversation because it is polite and because I thought the thin girl, the one I was interested in, would appreciate my sensitivity.

During the conversation, it quickly became apparent that the bigger girl was friendlier and that we had some common interests. The thin girl wasn't interested in what I was saying or what I looked like—which meant she wasn't interested in me. When the bigger girl asked me to dance, I hesitated at first. But I quickly sized up the situation. I was going nowhere with the thin girl. So I went dancing.

Immediately, I discovered something about this bigger girl. She could move. She was liquid. It turns out that she had been a cheerleader at the University of Pittsburgh. We both were readers and she enjoyed the poetry I recited in her ear. The eight bottles of beer I drank added to my attraction to her.

I ended up back at her apartment. Part of the conversation went to the subjects of nutrition and fitness. She was fit. There was no doubt about that. But, like many females, she was overly concerned about her body type, most of which was not in her control. She mentioned to me that she was seeing a psychologist for assistance with weight control—not to help her be more comfortable in the body her parents gave her but to help her lose weight. While she was bigger, she was lean. I didn't know where the weight loss would come from. On her refrigerator door, she had written a note to herself, "Don't put any fat in your body." The note was placed there as a suggestion from the psychologist.

The girl had a copy of a book titled *Stop the Insanity!* by Susan Powter. If you don't know the name, Powter was one of many nutrition and fitness "experts" who come and go on a regular basis. Her "thing" was that she had an interesting look— platinum flat-top haircut and a flat stomach (which her brother later claimed was the result of plastic surgery). She had an aggressive demeanor in her infomercials and got play on the talk shows of the day. I picked up the book and, in two hours, finished it. It was similar to eating a high-calorie but totally unsatisfying meal. Nothing of substance. Powter, like the psychologist, thought fat was the enemy and railed against eating fat. She was loud—and wrong.

Fat is your friend. Eating fat cuts calories. Eating fat promotes blood sugar regulation. Fat provides satiety. The consumption of dietary fat may result in a better hormonal balance. Fat is good for you...but that's not always been the case *(not from a physiological aspect but from a political one)*.

In 1977, Senator George McGovern chaired a committee, Dietary Goals for the United States. Using questionable science, and probably having some economic and political influence, the committee decided that the best diet for all was one that was low in fat and high in carbohydrates. Some of the questionable science used was an often-quoted 1958 study conducted by Ancel Keys, the Seven Countries Study. The purpose of Keys' study was to find a correlation between cardiovascular disease and diet. For years, this study was cited often when discussing the importance of low-fat diets and a reduction in heart disease. But, upon further review, it was revealed that Keys "cherry picked" the countries included in the study and ignored countries whose epidemiology was contrary to his results. Most notably, two countries that have high fat consumption, The Netherlands and Norway, have low rates of heart disease but were left out of the study. Inversely, a country with low fat consumption and high rates of heart disease, Chile, was left out also.

When Senator McGovern's committee released its report the food industry started turning out low-fat products—as they should have—and the talk shows of the day featured low-fat, high-carbohydrate gurus to tout the message. The only problem: it didn't work. On a note of irony and bad science, the U.S. obesity level started to climb after the committee's report was released. From a level of 15% in 1980, the obesity rate rose to 31% in 2000. The government told us how to eat, the food industry made the products based on the government's recommendation, and what was the result? America got fatter.

It wasn't until July of 2002 that good science got in the way of bad science. The *New York Times* published an article by science journalist Gary Taubes titled, "What If It's All Been a Big Fat Lie?" This was the first shot against the low-fat, high-carbohydrate thinking. Taubes referenced the bad science used in the McGovern report.

Since then, a number of articles and studies have given support to Taubes' work. I have a copy of a *Wall Street Journal* article from the May 3 – 4, 2014 weekend edition titled "Fat (Reconsidered)." One of the amazing points the author makes is that the American Heart Association (AHA) was a struggling non-profit in 1948. Procter & Gamble was promoting a new product and made the AHA the beneficiary of the marketing project. The new product launch raised $1.7 million for the AHA and set it on the road to the large non-profit, revenue-generating group it is today. The new product? Crisco. The ultimate provider of unfriendly trans-fatty acids for decades, until a formula change in 2007.

When I returned to the nutrition trade, I met with much resistance from the Nutrition Advice Industry. Instead of trying to determine if I had anything of value to offer, the NAI did what they could to prevent me from presenting free seminars. I remember one dance with a person who had an MS in Health Sciences who had never heard of Gary Taubes until I told her about him. Taube's seminal NYT article appeared in 2002, the conversation occurred in early 2014. The NAI has been slow to see the "fat" light. In addition to not appreciating what objective science writers were presenting about fat, they didn't give attention to a book published early in 2014 that should have been introduced by the NAI to the general public. The title of the book was, *The Big Fat*

Surprise: Why Butter, Meat and Cheese Belong in a Healthy Diet. The author was Nina Teicholz, an investigative journalist with an educational background in biology and an impressive writing CV. The length of her book may have been a turn-off to the NAI (along with an American public with "shrinking attention spans" looking for quick fixes through magazines supported by advertisers and puff piece internet articles). A serious study of nutrition advice over the last few decades was important to me, should have been important to you, but wasn't important to the NAI.

What does Number 20 mean to you? It means you have to start incorporating healthy, appetite suppressing fats into your diet. If you eat fish for the Omega-3s, then you need to eat olive oil for the Omega-9s and coconut oil for the appetite satisfying saturated fat (a bogeyman no longer; there are over 50 different types of saturated fat). Coconut oil has become a favorite of the ketogenic diet crew (minimal carbohydrate), bodybuilders, and myself. Essential fatty acids replace empty carbohydrate calories, can satisfy between-meal hunger pangs and provide a great source of medium chain triglycerides (MCTs). Most oils consist of long-chain triglycerides (LCTs). Soybean oil, for instance, is 100% LCTs. Coconut oil is 60% MCTs. MCTs are immediate sources of fuel as they travel directly from the intestinal tract to the liver. Less of the coconut oil is left to circulate through the body. Back in my darkest days when I sold body-building supplements, MCTs were a popular item among body builders in their never-ending quest to get bigger.

Coconut oil is solid at room temperature. I use it to marinate, as a salad dressing, and I've sautéed with the oil. On occasion, when my 2:00 p.m. hunger hits, I've taken a half teaspoon of coconut oil from the jar directly. It has a sweet taste and, due to its incredibly low ranking on the Glycemic Index, provides extended satiety.

I have a client in a wheelchair. He uses coconut oil to prevent skin sores. Females I've talked to say they use it on their skin. On occasion, I've put it in my hair before getting into a chlorine-rich swimming pool.

In closing this section, I want to share that I have mixed emotions when discussing healthy fats and their importance in calorie cutting. When I started reading nutrition books, among the first books I read were the Pritikin diet books. If you don't know the story, Nathan Pritikin was a chemical engineer and inventor who was diagnosed with heart disease in 1957. He became his own epidemiologist and studied cultures around the world with low rates of heart disease and cancer. He determined that the diet used by these cultures—low in fat and high in unrefined complex carbohydrates—was the diet for individuals looking to reverse heart disease and reduce their weight. The Pritikin books spawned the Pritikin Longevity Centers, where participants live the lifestyle for one or two weeks, learning low-fat cooking, and stress reduction techniques— everything they need to know to follow this diet when they return home.

I thought Pritikin was the answer as to how most of us should eat. But when I read *Beyond Pritikin* by Ann Louis Gittleman, my thought process started to change. Ms. Gittleman had been employed at the Pritikin Center and objected to their extremely low-fat diet. Ms. Gittleman's book touted the health benefits of healthy fats and how to cook with fats. As I started to put this document together, I realized there are people who will reduce/eliminate carbohydrate calories (mostly refined) if they incorporate healthy fats in their diet. And this is contrary to the original Pritikin message.

The same goes for Dean Ornish, M.D. Dr. Ornish has produced impressive results with controlled studies showing individuals with coronary heart disease can reverse their stenosis when following his diet, meditation, exercise programming. Like Pritikin, Ornish promotes an extremely low-fat diet. My personal compromise with suggesting that healthy fats can decrease overall calorie consumption, while knowing low-fat providers such as Pritikin and Ornish have impressive results, is this: nutrition is not an exact science. One person may benefit from a vegetarian diet; it may kill that person's twin brother. You may thrive on the Pritikin diet; your best friend may struggle with it. I may do great on the Paleo diet, you may object to the animal protein consumption. There is some combination of factors that will enable you to thrive on a certain diet while I fade on the same diet. The point is to find the food combination and eating habits that will enable you to thrive while reducing your calorie consumption.

At the end of the section on fiber, I shared the fact that I ate an avocado while writing it. In addition to the 6 grams of fiber, that same avocado also contained a healthy dose (20 grams) of monounsaturated fat. A year and a half ago, I never even had an avocado in my hand. Now I eat them multiple times during the week.

Number 21 Pay Homage to Desserts
You may think it odd, a section on desserts in a book detailing ways to cut calories, but hear me out. There has been cake and pie in the world long before we had the issue with obesity and diet-related Type II diabetes. A piece of Boston crème pie or cherry pie with coffee after dinner is not the culprit. The culprit is found in other sections of this document.

Let's imagine this: dinner is over. You've eaten a healthy meal with appropriate portions. You paid attention to Hara Hachi Bu, you didn't have the serving pot in front of you and autonomously grab seconds, and you didn't overconsume alcohol to lower your impulse control. You incorporated fiber into your meal. You did a good job at dinner. So have dessert! You're done eating for the night. In Europe, dessert signals the end of the meal. Here, for many, it signals the beginning of the grazing period. Going forward, don't be afraid of your dessert but use it as a celebration of a meal well done and a period of not eating until the next day. I eat apple/cherry pie with coffee on a regular basis. I have used the zero calorie Cool-Whip with strawberries as a dessert.

While I was preparing this document, a study was released discussing the concept of eating bread at the end of a meal. The participants, Type II diabetics, were able to better control glucose when using bread at the end of a meal, almost as a dessert. If you buy into the concept that the refined wheat in bread creates havoc with blood sugar, whole grain bread and butter for dessert may be a prudent idea.

Number 22 Snacks

The Institutes of Medicine (IOM) arrives at the 2,000 calorie per day diet by allotting you three meals with 640 calories each and two snacks with 80 calories each. Adjustments are made for activity level, age, and Resting Metabolic Rate (RMR). Eighty calories can go by in a New York minute. One Reese's Peanut Butter Cup is 105 calories (not the entire package—one cup!). My way to look at a snack: make it like a planned event. Don't think of snacks as something to have whenever the mood strikes you throughout the day or you come across a "food moment" (advertisement in a store, on a billboard, store signage). Plan your snacks, don't use them to graze. Think of snacks that require a knife and fork. I use pinto beans, red cabbage, and honey mustard as a snack. Same with avocado and black beans. Black beans and lime juice is an easy snack to prepare. I've also used oatmeal for a snack, as well as tuna and bean combinations. Try to get away from traditional "hand" snacks (chips, cookies, etc.) Two cool hand snacks—frozen grapes and raw corn on the cob. Put a container of washed green grapes in the freezer. The combination of crispness, sweetness, and cold makes for a filling snack. Before trying the raw corn on the cob, I thought the kernels would have been tough to chew. I was 100% wrong. The "mouthfeel" is sweet, tasty, juicy, and makes for a great midday snack.

Number 23 Brush Your Teeth Immediately after Eating

This is a trick used by high school and college wrestlers who have to watch their weight during the season. Right after eating, brush your teeth. Prevents grazing. Like enjoying your fine dessert, you are recognizing that the meal is over.

Number 24 "Intermittent" Fasting

While the act of fasting is common in certain religions as a means to cleanse the soul, intermittent fasting may provide benefits for the rest of the body. You know all those antioxidant supplements sold in the health food store? They're marketed as a way to diffuse free radicals. Where do the free radicals come from? From the process of eating and digesting food. Intermittent fasting (maybe skipping a few meals or limiting food intake one to three days per week) would limit free radical production and provide other benefits. From *Scientific American:*

"...occasional fasting increases the level of

"chaperone proteins," which prevent the incorrect assembly of other molecules in the cell. Additionally, fasting mice have higher levels of brain-derived neurotrophic factor (BDNF), a protein that prevents stressed neurons from dying. Low levels of BDNF have been linked to everything from depression to Alzheimer's, although it is still unclear whether these findings reflect cause and effect. Fasting also ramps up autophagy, a kind of garbage-disposal system in cells that gets rid of damaged molecules, including ones that have been previously tied to Alzheimer's, Parkinson's, and other neurological diseases." (Scientific American; Special Collector's Edition, Volume 24, Number 1).

The author of this piece also discussed the fact that intermittent fasting's main effect seems to be increasing the body's responsiveness to insulin. Decreased sensitivity to insulin often accompanies obesity and has been linked to diabetes and heart failure.

What is this type of fasting? To me, we can pick our spots as to when we fast. You can plan in advance which day you'll fast or have an extremely low-calorie day. Do that once per week. You can have a lunch, not have dinner, and have a light snack late at night. You can eat a full dinner (with dessert!) and not eat again until the morning. You may choose to fast on a day where you're not at your stressful job and will have an easier time of defeating your impulses to eat. A great time to fast may be in the morning. The concept of three meals a day with snacks in between is a relatively new concept in the history of humans. Abundance of food is new; periods of scarcity were the rule for a much longer period. We've been told since day one in kindergarten that breakfast is the most important meal of the day. I am going to respectfully disagree with that adage and say "the first meal of the day is the most important one." Don't feel the need to eat just because it's morning. I have had breakfast when I was not hungry but ate out of routine. It was the act of eating that made me hungry. What I ate caused my blood sugar to increase and then, due to the insulin response, decrease. I then was on the vicious cycle in search of easy to get refined carbohydrates to give me the energy to get through the day. Those days when I woke up not hungry, I could have benefitted by having my first meal until later in the day.

An idea: why not try to fast for 10 to 12 hours from your last meal of the evening to your "break fast" the next day? That will give you a half a day with no food to allow your body's blood sugar and insulin to do what they're supposed to do.

One key note about fasting: it is important to plan your "breaking fast" meal, regardless of when you are having that meal. Plan it in advance. One of my Muslim friends, when fasting during Ramadan, has evening meals planned for his family on each of the fasting days.

Number 25 Exercise Does Not Give a Reason to Overconsume

Most people overestimate the amount of calories exercise utilizes. The average person utilizes 80 to 100 calories per hour due to normal functions. This is known as the Resting Metabolic Rate (RMR). When you read calorie counts per hour for exercises or on machines, the RMR is included in the amount. And the longer you do an exercise, the more your body gets acclimated to it, and therefore the fewer calories it uses. Don't overeat after an exercise session and justify it to yourself by thinking that you expended more calories than you're about to consume. You have to plan your post-workout meals.

I have the perfect story for this section. When I became a fitness swimmer, there was a time when swimming a mile was still a challenge for me. On a Saturday afternoon one summer, I drove to the Oliver Bath House (OBH) in the South Side of Pittsburgh. I was living in the neighborhood of Baldwin at the time. OBH is a 20-yard pool. I swam 88 lengths to complete the one-mile swim. I showered, got dressed, and left the building. I had one of those intense post-swimming hungers. (I no longer get that type of hunger after swimming.)

A few blocks away on Carson Street, Ron's Pizza Palace called my name. I stopped in for a few slices. Farther up Carson, I noticed that The Pretzel Shop was still open. I stopped in for a couple of pretzels and, probably, a chocolate milk. As I was turning from Carson onto Becks Run Road, there was no line at Page's Dairy Mart. No line at Page's is a rare treat. I don't remember what I had, but I certainly stopped for ice cream. And I'm sure I ate something else as soon as I walked in the house.

How many calories did I use swimming one mile in a 20-yard pool? The internet says about 400. (300 more than if I didn't swim but sat around in the house). And how many calories did I consume after swimming? A lot more than 400—maybe 4,000.

On a related note: my swims are generally early in the a.m. For the longest time, I would eat before swimming. Shredded Wheat or generic Cheerios with rice milk or microwaved oatmeal. I would eat again after returning from the pool. About three years ago, I decided not to eat before swimming. As my swims are about one mile, I was concerned that I wouldn't have the energy to complete the swim. To my surprise, it didn't make a difference. As of this writing, I am swimming longer distances, have added interval training, and my lack of food before swimming has been a benefit. If you think about it, if I swim five times per week, I may have eliminated 1,000 to 1,500 calories per week.

Final note: fasting, not eating before working out, and limiting your calorie consumption after working out may assist you in converting your "stored energy" into glucose.   We all are carrying calories in our midsection. You may see it as unsightly fat but you have to appreciate the fact that if your ancestors didn't have the ability to store that fat, you wouldn't be here today. When you are utilizing energy without consuming it, the hormone glucagon does the opposite of insulin. It works to convert stored fat to glucose.

As I write this, there is a chiropractor who advertises on a local radio show. He holds himself out to be a "weight loss expert" (this year's version of Susan Powter). His sponsored programming and ads tout fat "melting away." He doesn't bother to share with the unsuspecting and unsophisticated audience that this is a physiological impossibility. The way one loses weight is to get into their fat stores, have the calories converted to glucose, utilized, and then not replaced. But there is not enough revenue generated by that simple statement to buy advertising time and pay for sponsored programming to share that information.

Number 26 **Get the Sleep Your Body and Mind Needs**

If you don't get enough sleep, you will spend your day (or your brain will spend the day) in search of easy-to-digest carbohydrates. Proper sleep will aid in "ungrazing" (not really a word, I know). You may start the day off on the wrong foot by eating a highly refined breakfast. If I were to start the day off with Cinnamon French toast, a staple in my household growing up, the rest of the day would be spent fighting to stay alert and in search of carbohydrates.

If you have to give up watching the Channel 11 News to get to bed earlier, so be it. There isn't anything on that broadcast that a 30-second search of the internet can't find. The local news in my city is ten minutes of news, four minutes of weather, three minutes of conversation about the local football team (even during the offseason), two minutes of happy banter between the anchors, and eight minutes of commercials, one human interest story, and the slickly-produced introduction and sign-off.

Sleep experts will tell you that to promote healthy sleep, don't use your bed as a desk, TV watching platform or place to eat. Early in the evening, you should make sure you bed is clear of clothes, books, etc. Go into your sleep area a few hours before sleep, turn the bed cover down, and put on a soft nightlight. Make your bed an inviting place. When you sleep, leave your technology somewhere else. Many of us use our phones as alarm clocks. Don't do that. Leave your main phone in another room. Use a second phone for the alarm or—shocking idea—how about an actual alarm clock or clock radio? I have a clock radio next to the bed. If I wake up in the middle of the night, I put the radio on for "sleep" mode and listen to an all-night light subject conversation talk show. I tend to go back to sleep easily. For those few nights when I wake up and can't get back to sleep, I go to another room and always have a book waiting. A few minutes of reading advances my place in the book and helps me return to sleep.

Sleep experts will also tell you that the idea of "catching up" with your sleep over the weekend does not work. You can't be sleep deprived during the week and sleep multiple hours over the weekend and be even. Two negatives, in this case, do not a positive make. At the time of this writing, I wake up at 4 a.m. to go swimming at 5 a.m. There is one day that seems to occur once every two weeks when I wake up and I realize that my body needs sleep more than it needs to swim. I go back to sleep and have the deepest, most restful sleep over the next two hours with some of the most vivid dreams imaginable. *(How about a walk around the neighborhood before bed or a bike ride? When I started swimming my pool stayed open until ten p.m. I had some great late-night swims and even greater, deeper sleep sessions after).*

Sleep well and you will reduce your calories.

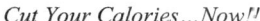

"One cannot think well, love well, sleep well, if one has not dined well."

-- Virginia Woolf

PART THREE: THE MENTAL ASPECTS OF CALORIE CUTTING

Number 27 Control Those Impulses—*Or They Will Control You!!*

This is the most important factor in cutting your calories. We teased it in a few spots but we've waited until now to present it. It involves your brain—an organ more important than your stomach when it comes to consuming calories.

Think back to the glorious days before home food delivery service, a pizza joint on every other corner, hundreds of different corporate restaurant chains, supermarkets and convenience stores. Hard for us to imagine but there was a time when it was actually difficult to obtain food. But that time existed. And our brains, which utilize 20% to 25% of daily calories consumed, became wired to be on the lookout for food, especially easy-to-digest calories. You—in the form of your brain—didn't know when food would be available next.

If you think you have weak willpower, think about this: you have the willpower to get up in the morning, go to a job, do that job, go home and take care of your children, your spouse, and, in some cases, your parents. You have the willpower to get to a gym three times per week and, perhaps, a religious facility of your choice once or more per week. You have the willpower to do those things. That craving for food is not lack of willpower—it's evolutionary adaptation.

This is not an excuse to spend the day motoring through the drive-through lane at fast food restaurants, stopping in at convenience stores to buy impulse items or raiding the refrigerator at night. **In**

essence, our brains have not evolved to handle the overabundance of food available to most of us. But don't blame evolution for your desire for food. Other factors are at play.

While the impulse to eat is hard wired in us, we also do things to decrease the impulse control we do have. Alcohol consumption, exposing ourselves to too many "impulse challenges" (you'll eventually lose some of them), forgetting H.A.L.T.S. (see Number 12), and being fatigued (see Number 26) will lead to overconsumption of calories. Do you have a dog? What do you do when your dog yawns? Same thing happens when somebody tells you they're starving and asks if you want to get "something to eat." You forget about Number 12 and tend to agree with them.

The main thing you can do to control your impulses—and this may be the most important part of this document—is to PLAN YOUR MEALS & YOUR SNACKS. If you have a family, you should be giving some thought to your meal planning for the week. You can fine-tune this plan each morning by writing down the meals and snacks you'll have for the day and, if possible, at what time you'll eat them. This is the opposite of the inefficient food journals where individuals are asked to write everything they've eaten. The studies I've read reveal that people underreport, forget to list between-meal snacks, etc. But writing down your meals and snacks in advance would have a different result.

Impulse control also has an important role in behavioral finance. It is important for an individual to be able to control impulse purchases for items other than that Reese's Peanut Butter Cup at the checkout line. Your ability to control impulse purchases is a major factor in predicting your future financial health. I read a story about a man who developed a great way to control his impulse purchases. If he saw an item he wanted to buy, and that item cost more than $250, he would return home and write the product and price in a notebook. Thirty days later, if he still wanted to buy it, he did. But what happened to him typically was that he would come across a different impulse item that replaced the previous one on the list. The item he wanted more started the new 30-day countdown over again. If you're going to follow that plan, pick a dollar amount that fits in prudently with your budget.

Number 28 *The Economist* Article

When I was going back through my crate full of nutrition/fitness articles and notes I had compiled over the years, I came across an article from *The Economist* titled "Mild and bitter: The evolutionary origin of depression." (June 25, 2009). If you don't know this magazine, it is one of the greatest magazines in the world. It is published in England and provides insight into American business and society that U.S.-based publications can't deliver. The magazine also writes on social science topics that regular business periodicals don't. I subscribed to this magazine when I thought it was a monthly. It was a bittersweet moment when I found it was weekly. The material is first rate;on a weekly basis it was too much to blend in with all the other reading I have to do. I now read it only when the cover jumps out at me.

When I saw the "Mild and bitter" article I was puzzled as to why I put it in my crate related to nutrition and fitness. I reread it and realized why I deemed it important enough "crate" it. The author cites work done by Randolph Neese, a psychologist and researcher in evolutionary medicine at the University of Michigan. Dr. Neese's observation is that a percentage of the population suffers from "low mood." Low mood is a protective device to keep that percentage of the population with low mood from doing psychological damage by "pursuing unreachable goals." The author explains in the same way that mild pain prevents you from doing an activity and causing further pain, there is a percentage of the population that realizes their goals and ambitions are too lofty and low mood stops their pursuit in order to prevent "mind damage" (my quote).

I'm an extremely ambitious person. But my creative pursuits haven't been met. I've had exciting experiences and insights and have created some interesting things. But what I set out to achieve has gone unmet. That hasn't stopped me from continuing to pursue my ambitions. There have been different costs paid for not giving up ambition. The idea that I had to go into the basement of an old shoe store and sell bodybuilding supplements—after obtaining the level of knowledge I did in the areas of nutrition and fitness—is a perfect example.

One of those costs has been, at times, the over-consumption of food. And, most often, not the high-fiber, high-phytonutrient, low-sugar, low-refined carbohydrate food that would have served me best.

Just knowing that Dr. Neese's concept exists has provided me the insight to deal with "lack of creation eating" (again, my quote). This insight may help you as well, but it may not help others. If you are an ambitious, creative soul, we're kindred spirits. But not everybody shares our need to create, achieve, and accomplish, and not everybody has ambition. So Number 26 will not be a calorie-cutting method for all of us. Just you and me.

In closing, I constantly tell people that my middle name is "Persistence." In the article, the author makes the comment that "Persistence, though necessary for success and considered a virtue by many, can also have a negative impact on health." I seriously doubt that if I would have read this article 20 years ago that my middle name would be any different.

Number 29 **Find the Point to Your Life**

Many years ago, I was transferring my investment license from one firm to another. There was a delay in the transfer and I was out of the business for a few months. Because I had both real estate and banking experience, a person I knew who worked for a mortgage company asked me to come to work for him as a temporary employee. The operation was in a large building in the North Side of Pittsburgh. My specific job was to work with the home builders, their customers, and the lender's inspectors to authorize the release of "draws" during the construction process. Going in, I knew the builders would be asking for draws on work that hadn't been completed yet. I had heard similar whining before.

Even though I was there for a short period of time, it was a horrible existence. Most of the people who worked in this company were content to toil in a low-paying job with minimal opportunity for advancement. There were also a number of banking "lifers" who were, like me, now working as temps. They wore the suits they wore to PNC, Mellon, and Equibank twenty years before, read the *Wall Street Journal* and tried to sound intelligent discussing the movement of the stock market and specific stocks— in between the time they were making copies and sending faxes.

There was one thing that kept me stable and sane during this experience. We were close to a shopping area with a well-known fast food franchise. Like a zombie, each day at noon I walked like one of the living dead to this restaurant. I ordered the same thing every day. I always got double tomatoes on my hamburger, thinking that was a healthy thing to do.

I couldn't wait to bite into those trans-fatty acid-rich French fries and feel the grease slide down the back of my throat. That thick burger was great and would have been great even without the extra tomato. The rich chocolate drink that finished the meal got me through a few hours of the afternoon. I know now that eating those meals created brain chemicals (endorphins, dopamine, enkephalins, etc.) that gave me a few moments reprieve from my dull daily existence.

There were days that I would leave this job, go home, eat a pizza, and go right to bed. It was a depressing existence.

How is my story going to help you cut calories? Easy. Find the point to your life. Do what needs to be done so you don't have to spend the morning waiting for the big and little hands to reach twelve so you can do the zombie walk to the fast food joint. If this means spending your evenings and weekends learning new job skills, developing a business while holding down a full-time job, so be it. It this means not spending Sundays watching pro football most of the day, so be it. I knew what the point to my life was when I did this job. It was just a hurdle on the journey. In hindsight, I wish I would have handed my period of severe underemployment better than I did. I wish I didn't make the bad nutrition choices I did.

I know many people will read the last two sections and identity with me. They will tell themselves that they overeat because their ambitions haven't been met. But you know what? Somebody has to be the "jagoff" (popular Pittsburgh term). I have learned this over the years: when you're the person who stands up and says "I want to create, achieve and accomplish," there will be jagoffs on the other side of the table who will stand up and say, "Not on my watch." They will do things to block your path toward creativity. Their form of creating is blocking you from creating. As I write this, I think about the tenacity that certain members of the Nutrition Advice Industry exhibited, going out of their way to prevent me from doing free seminars and discussing my adventures in the nutrition trade. I will admit that they won the battle. I overconsumed food—unhealthy food choices—during that time. But they lost the war. This document wouldn't have been created without their "help."

Number 30 Eudora Welty's and Norman Drabble's Contributions to This Document

This one is probably the only time in the history of the written word that a famous American short story writer will be discussed along with a great American comic strip character.

I became aware of Eudora Welty when I was studying literature at community college. She was a writer from Mississippi and excelled at the short story format. One of her pieces of advice to writers was to finish a day of writing knowing exactly where you'll start the next day. Finishing a day of writing not knowing where you'll pick up the next day is sheer anguish.

I will make this short leap: if possible, finish up a day of work knowing exactly how you'll start the next day. The uncertainty may cause overconsumption at dinner, after dinner and at breakfast. Pay special attention to your Monday morning starting point. A weekend spent wondering about your Monday morning assignments may lead to "over-ing" (new word) during the weekend (over-eating, over-drinking).

I'm a major fan of the comic strip *Drabble*. When I ask people if they read it, most people answer in the negative. I'm amazed at how many adults do not read the comics section of the newspaper. Norman

Drabble has been a community college student since I started reading the strip. As a one-time community college student, I have a connection to Norman. His father, Ralph, is a mall guard and doughnut expert. One of the memorable episodes was when Ralph explained how the mall guard nightstick could be used for many things—and then showed us a stack of doughnuts being carried on his nightstick.

In a recent *Drabble*, Ralph told his wife, Honeybunch, how much he hated Thursdays. When she asked "Why?" he replied, "Because on Thursdays I start thinking about how much I hate Mondays." I used to have a job where on Sunday afternoon I would start dreading having to go to work on Monday. I was underemployed and worked with a bunch of folks who only cared about what they were going to watch on TV that night and how the local football team would do the coming Sunday. My ambition and desire to create, matched with a boring job, resulted in many poor food choices.

Among the points to be made in this section: if you're not a daily reader of the comics, become one. You don't even have to get a newspaper. The comics are available through many sources on the internet. An investment of five minutes per day reading the comics provides an invaluable return on that time. Reading the comics won't cut calories but you'll be a happier person.

Number 31 Reinforce Your Nutrition Education with Ongoing and Objective Information

Any educator will tell you that the reinforcement of what is taught is as important as the subject matter. When I started my process of reading nutrition books, attending seminars, and interviewing nutritionists, I developed a reading list of magazines. Most of the magazines I read (*University of California at Berkley Wellness*

Newsletter, Tufts Health & Nutrition Letter, and
Nutrition Action Newsletter, among others) were
"advertiser-free." The editors/writers didn't have to
worry about ticking off an advertiser. Therefore, they
were able to provide objective, science-based
information. Reading these monthly newsletters
provided me with knowledge of nutrition and fitness
topics and reinforcement of that knowledge,
sometimes in the same issue.

One ad-sponsored magazine I remember fondly
was *Longevity.* The publisher, Kathy Keeton, was a
survivor of childhood polio who later became a
stripper, actress and, eventually, the wife of
Penthouse magazine publisher Bob Guccione. Ms.
Keeton had developed an interest in the subject of
anti-aging. When I first got into her magazine, I
thought it was one of the best advertiser-supported
magazines of its kind. But as time went on, the
editorial content started to change. The types of ads
changed also. It seemed that an article on a topic
would be followed, eight pages later, with an
advertisement for a product connected to that article.
My theory? The cost of publishing a professional
magazine probably overtook the luxury of being
objective and the articles had to become more
"advertiser-friendly" to keep publishing.

I believe the magazine faded away a few years
before Ms. Keeton passed away in 1997.

Now I read my nutrition/fitness/lifestyle
publications online. The American Council on
Science and Health (ACSH) publishes a daily
"Dispatch" delivered into my inbox. Four or five
articles on a timely topic presented in the Council's
creed: "Science. Not Hype." The ACSH provides insightful work on the supplement industry, the anti-
vaccine movement, GMOs, etc. I also read a blog
presented by Marion Nestle, PhD, MPH. Dr. Nestle
(ironic name for doing what she does) is the author of

Why Calories Count: From Science to Politics, and *Food Politics: How the Food Industry Influences Nutrition & Health*. The title of the last book is also the name of Dr. Nestle's blog. Dr. Stephen Barrett, the quack's worst nightmare, publishes an electronic newsletter titled *Consumer Health Digest*. Dr. Barrett reports on legal action against sellers of supplements, providers of illicit, unproven cancer treatments, and those trying to separate the misinformed and unhealthy from their money.

These daily nutrition and health blogs are available to you. Get to the respective sites and sign up using your email address. The objectivity of the ACSH and Dr. Nestle will help you in numerous ways. ACSH, Stephen Barrett and Marion Nestle produce some of the most insightful articles on nutrition. And none of them are part of the NAI.

Number 32 Think of Calories in Three-Day Periods

I think there have been millions of people who have, millions of times, started a dietary program under their own definition of "healthy eating" only to be waylaid by a restaurant meal, a social/business event, year-end holidays, vacation, or something that caused them to drop their impulse control. Instead of getting right back on that definition of healthy eating (whatever their own definition is), they gave up the ghost and returned to their regular eating routine.

If you take the calorie-cutting methods listed here and apply them to your nutritional habits, don't worry if you overconsume one day or over a weekend. Instead, think of your calorie consumption over a three-day period. If you know you're attending a social/business event where alcohol and food will be served, use the day before or after as one of your intermittent fasting days. Pay attention to your alcohol consumption, go for fiber in your food selection, and don't let a day of overeating derail you. Get back on track the next day.

One related note: When I was putting my presentation together in early 2014, I started eating the way defined in this document. My weight decreased in a short period by 18 pounds. People were commenting on my weight loss. And I'll be honest: those words felt good. But when my weight loss plateaued, those words stopped. And it made me wonder how many people cut their calories, increased their physical activity, started to lose weight, got the compliments, bought the smaller clothes, and then, when the words of praise stopped, returned to their previous eating habits? In my case, when I saw somebody I hadn't seen in a while and they *didn't* make a comment about my weight loss, I felt slighted. And that was silly! I wasn't eating differently to lose weight. I was just applying the calorie-cutting techniques being shared in this document.

Number 33 Appreciate the Correlation between Writing and Being Hungry

Here is a quick class on writing. The process of writing is not like what you see on TV or in movies. There is never a garbage can with dozens of crumpled-up sheets in and around the can. There is not an ashtray full of ashes and cigarette butts on the desk. Most of the writing process takes place away from the computer or typewriter (the first things I wrote of any length were done on a Smith-Corona electric typewriter which I still have). Writing is thinking about the subject matter, how you will begin, the points you want to make, and an ending that brings everything together. Your subconscious is doing the heavy lifting at first.

If you are writing a screenplay, the thinking

process includes a visual beginning, developing the characters, the dialogue, the subplots, the set-ups, the transitions, the plot points, how the romantic interests will meet, the climax and a satisfying ending. Before literally writing the script, an outline must be structured. You may get to a point where you have gotten your main character up a tree and rocks are being thrown at him. You have to figure out how to get him down from that tree. While your subconscious has gotten you to this point, there is a moment when you will have to sit down and do "focused brainstorming" to keep the story moving. You will have to come up with an idea that is plausible, that fits in with what has already been presented and that you can connect the rest of the story to. In the same vein, if you write you will, at some point, develop writer's block. You can walk away from the project for a period, turn your attention to another project, or do what seasoned writers do—push your way through. Put something on the paper. It is easier to clean up something already written than to put something down when you have the block.

So how does this shortened writing class pertain to eating? There will be times when you are 1.5 to 2 hours away from a meal. And you're hungry. You're just going to have to suck it up and tough it out. No other way to explain it. You may be able to drop into a convenience store, go to the candy machine, or drive through a takeout window, but you don't want to do that. If you've planned your meals and snacks for the day and you've got hunger pangs, you should do what I do—enjoy the feeling of being hungry! Many Americans haven't felt true hunger for a long time. At the slightest feeling of stomach or mouth hunger, they're caving in. Enjoy a growling stomach. It's a sign that you are gaining control of your calorie consumption.

Number 34 Surround Yourself with Visions of Healthy Food

In your kitchen, hang framed prints or drawings of healthy, appetizing food. In my kitchen I have a beautiful print of onions. There are Vidalia, yellow, red, and white onions. In the foreground, there is a cutting board with slices of the onion varieties. In the background, whole onions are waiting their turn on the board. I had the print professionally framed. I see the picture both consciously and subliminally throughout the day. My theory is that being exposed to healthy photos of food may lead you to make healthier food choices, lower-calorie ones, instead of high-calorie, only momentarily satisfying ones. You can visit galleries to see if local artists have produced any paintings showing healthy food combinations or have an artist custom-make a painting to your order. There are also websites you can visit to acquire prints. When you acquire your "food art" get the print professionally framed. It makes a major difference in the final presentation. *NOTE: There are zero fried onion rings in my beautiful picture.*

Did you know: There are over 150 phytonutrients in an onion, including "quercetin" (kwur-si-tin). In my files, I have an undated note referencing a past issue of *Gastroenterology,* which states that quercetin helps prevent the bacterium responsible for many types of cancer.

Number 35 Practice "Mindful Munching"

Many years ago, before I entered the investment business, I was involved in various ventures and had various jobs. I had a temporary job with the U.S. Census Bureau. My job was to go into the city of Clairton, Pennsylvania and do two things: locate the people who the previous Census taker had missed and determine the fate of certain housing units. At the time, Clairton did not have a police department and was considered a somewhat dangerous area. The only reason I got this job was because nobody else wanted it.

I had many interesting experiences in Clairton, a few of them slightly scary. All I had to protect myself was my U.S. Census Bureau I.D. badge (which many residents mistook for that of a parole officer) and my wits. I knocked many houses off the rolls. These houses were abandoned, rat-infested, and had no hope of being rehabbed.

There was one small area in town where the houses were nicely kept. I had started my job in the depressed part of town and was surprised to see this nice area. Because I needed to reach people at home, it was not uncommon for me to start my day after 4:00 p.m. One day I knocked on the door of a house in this "upscale" part of Clairton. The owners, a young couple, invited me in. These homes were older and small but this particular one was well kept. The couple was having their dinner. There were lit candles on the table and a half-full bottle of wine. Classical music was playing in the background. I thought to myself, "This was the way to have dinner." I didn't know it at the time but this couple was practicing what I know now as "mindful munching."

In our technology-driven lives, many of us are eating while reading, watching TV, replying to emails or talking with people while only paying half attention to the food we're shoveling into our mouths. The end result: we're missing the "full" signals and overconsuming calories.

Mindful munching is the art of not taking your food for granted, giving some thought to the long process it took to get to your table, turning off outside distractions, and concentrating on the texture, smell, appearance, and "mouthfeel" of the food.   Paying attention to our food, practicing meditative moments over it, will lead to reduced calorie consumption.

How can you practice Mindful Munching?

- Take a moment before eating to appreciate the fact you have the food and recognize the journey it took to get to you
- Turn off all distractions except for some classical music (to me, Sinatra counts as classical). If you are concentrating on a TV show or some technology, that will get more of your attention than the food.   This always results in overeating.
- Shut off your phone ringer. *On a semi-related note, many of the text messages you receive will have improved results if you don't reply to them ASAP. Time between texts is your friend.*
- Don't think about your dessert or next meal when eating the current one.   Focus on what is in front of you.   Appreciate what you have in the moment.

Two quotes for your review:

From Marc David's *Ordinary Magic: Everyday Life as Spiritual Path:*

Having dinner: Achieve the fullest experience of your food. Taste it. Savor it. Pay attention to it. Rejoice in it.   See how it makes your body feel. Take in all the sensations. But don't just eat the food. Eat the ambiance. Eat the colors. Eat the aromas. Eat the conversation. Eat the company sitting next to you. Eat the entire experience. We don't just hunger for food alone. We hunger for the experience of it—the tasting, the chewing, the sensuousness, the enjoyment, the textures, the sounds, and the satisfaction.

Marc David is the founder of the Institute for the Psychology of Eating *(If the name hadn't been taken, I would have used it.)* And remember this quote from an entity who knows something about mindfulness:

> *"Your body is precious. It is our vehicle for awakening. Treat it with care."*
> --Buddha

PART FOUR: THE SOCIAL & MEDIA ASPECTS OF CUTTING CALORIES

Number 36 Don't Be a "Food Pusher"

My grandmothers weren't career women. They weren't highly educated. My father's mother cleaned the bathrooms at the train station. My mother's mother helped her husband operate their combination pool room/poker den. Neither drove a car. But while neither had an impressive curriculum vitae (fancy word for résumé), they each possessed an amazing talent. They knew how to make food. My father's mother was Polish and my mother's mother was Serbian. You should be able to imagine the food I was exposed to as a child. My grandmothers wouldn't know the feeling of closing the big sale, getting the promotion with the new office or stock options (no pool room offers stock options), so they cooked and grilled and fried and baked. And they served. And when you were done eating, they suggested you eat some more. Their sense of creation and accomplishment came from preparing food and watching others enjoy it. Over the years, I have come across other Food Pushers (FP). I consumed far more food that I should have or wanted to at the insistence of these individuals. Part of the reason was that it was easy to twist my arm while sitting in front of serving platters of delicious food. The other reason was that I didn't want to hurt their feelings.

If you know a Food Pusher, let them know in gentle terms that you appreciate and respect their work but that you don't need to eat the amount of food they would want you to. Ask if you can take some of the food with you (often offered anyway) and make a meal or two over the next few days. If you are going to the home of a FP, maybe you can do an intermittent fast before or after the visit.

If you *are* a FP, please realize that the people in your life appreciate you for many things—not just your food expertise. Maybe you can concentrate on preparing lower-calorie, higher-fiber, more phyto-nutrient-dense meals than you have been making in the past.

One other family note: I had an uncle who was a child of the Depression. His wedding photo was in my grandparents' house. He was married in his Army uniform. Probably weighed 185 pounds on his wedding day. At the time of his death, he weighed over 400 pounds. He once rode in the front seat of my car. Every right turn resulted in the springs rubbing against the bottom of the fender. He told me there were many nights when he went to bed hungry as a kid. When he got to the point where food was available, he was going to make up for those hungry nights. When he got out of the Army, he got a job in a General Motors plant. He raised his six daughters, was a "ringer" for bowling teams and he ate. And ate.

I've heard similar stories of people who were deprived of food as a child doing things similar to my uncle. The famous actress Audrey Hepburn, though not of Dutch descent, spent WWII in Arnhem in the Netherlands. Her mother mistakenly thought the Netherlands would remain neutral during the war. The first clue her mother was wrong was when the Germans invaded the country. The Netherlands was subject to a "winter hunger" during 1944-1945. The Germans and the severe weather were the culprits. There was widespread starvation in the country and Ms. Hepburn had firsthand experience of living hungry.

When she became a working actress and achieved

both fame and fortune, it was reported that she kept canned goods stacked under her dining room table. She experienced hunger once and wasn't going to take the chance of repeating that experience. I'm sure there are many stories similar to my uncle's and Ms. Hepburn's.

Number 37 Don't Take Nutrition Advice from "They"

Many people make a statement to me— investment-related, nutrition-related, fitness-related —by telling me "They" say you should eat this/don't eat that/lift this way/don't lift this way/invest in this/stay away from that. I always ask them to give me the name and number of "They" because I want to call "They" and see where the information comes from. "They" seems to be an expert in everything.

What "You" don't realize is that "They" is a well-organized, well-capitalized marketing effort with the sole purpose of getting people to buy what "They" is selling. The businesses behind "They" have access to the media, the talk-show circuit, and your friends and associates. Businesses with products to sell have a vested interest in getting others to believe "They" know what they're talking about. And generally speaking, "They" don't.

Several of the best outlets for "They" to deliver messages are local newspapers/radio stations and TV stations. The assignment editors at these outlets like the simplistic messages "They" delivers because they need to deliver messages that the widest audience will be able to digest easily.

Eating nothing but cabbage soup will help you lose weight? That gets a mention on the six o'clock news. New pill in the works for weight loss? Definitely gets a story written. I write this with the full disclosure that the businesses I'm involved with require me to contact local media outlets with story suggestions and ideas. I've had 15 articles published in the local newspapers. I should have had 30 articles published based on the quality of what I submitted. I've been on radio shows discussing relevant, timely and topical subjects. I am an insightful and well-researched presenter. But it has been difficult for me to get booked on these shows because "They" has a more simplistic message or a connection to the broadcasting entity that is deemed more important than my objective, unbiased information.

Connected to Number 37, not deserving its own spot but important nonetheless: stop rationalizing your food choices. We've discussed not overeating because you'll "work it off" later. Other rationalizations: having a zero-calorie soda with a meal as a way to justify more calories, thinking the "thermogenic" burn of food you consume will result in negative calorie consumption or, my all-time favorite, the concept that birthday cake consumed on your birthday is calorie-free (Refer back to Number 21 to recall how I feel about birthday cake). If it's your birthday, enjoy a piece of cake. And don't feel the need to run two miles right after eating it to "burn it off" (whatever that means). The best way to eliminate rationalizing food: plan your meals and snacks. This will help with impulse control and eliminate rationalization.

To date, nobody has ever given me a phone number or email address for "They" and I don't expect to ever receive one.

Number 38 **Alcohol—"Less Is More"**

This title was used previously in a book to share the idea that, when out and about, drinking less alcohol will result in better control of your impulses, better control of your social skills; and a better time overall. I wrote about a friend of mine who over-consumed alcohol when we were out in clubs. He would order his second whiskey and water before finishing the first. Each successive drink would go down faster than the previous one. He was a good-looking guy, in shape, and he had money. Girls would "open" him with conversation. But he couldn't deal with any of them. The amount of alcohol, and the speed at which he drank it, interfered with his social skills. He couldn't conduct a conversation with any female. I would explain to him that he may be the coolest guy in town on three drinks but we would never find out because by the time that third drink would be circulating in his system, he already downed seven drinks.

According to Mark Bittman, *New York Times* writer, and prolific food author (*How to Cook Everything, Vegan Before 6 P.M., How to Cook Everything Fast*) alcohol calories are in the Top Five sources of calories for the typical American. The other four are baked goods, chicken, sugar-sweetened beverages, and pizza (Bittman was citing a U.S. Department of Agriculture (USDA) report.)

How many calories are there in alcohol? A bottle/can of regular beer has 154 calories; light beer has 96 calories. A five-ounce serving of wine (red or white) has about 125 calories per. If you were like my friend and enjoyed your whiskey, each shot is over 100 calories. If you do your drinking in social settings or at home, you can build up many calories in a relatively short period. Back in my ballroom days, I had many ten-bottle beer nights.

How can you reduce calories while still imbibing? Here are my suggestions:

1. Realize what I'm saying by "Less is more." You have that first drink and your impulse control has started to slide away.

2. Why finish a drink and order another immediately? That first drink may leave you with a cool buzz fifteen minutes from now. Let it do its work.

3. Don't consume alcohol two days in a row (tough to do at holiday time or while on vacation). If you have a "party" night in which you overdrink and overeat, refer back to Numbers 24 and 32. Do an intermittent fast after a night of heavy drinking/eating or include it in one of your "Three Day Periods."

The problem with alcohol, beyond the fast calories consumed, is that it lowers your impulse control. How many pizzas have we eaten after drinking beer? Too many to mention for me. Alcohol interferes with your sleep. Most of us pass out instead of falling asleep after a night of drinking and never get that great R.E.M. sleep we require. The next day, many times, becomes a "grazing" day when we keep eating in order to stay alert.

I will share this: I have been pulled over by police officers four times while under the influence of alcohol. I was legally intoxicated each time (and many times that I didn't get pulled over). I never got a Driving Under the Influence (DUI) citation. One would think I would have learned my lesson the first time, the second time, the third time or the fourth time. But my lesson wasn't learned until long after seeing the lights on the top of the police car in my review that fourth time. I just had too many birthdays and eventually realized all the costs involved with DUIs to try to navigate under the influence. Part of the lesson I learned is this: If you can't afford to take an Uber or taxi to get home after a night of drinking, you can't afford that night of drinking. A citation for a DUI has a much more ominous (and expensive) meaning today than it did when I was coming up.

I now enjoy being in locations where everybody is drinking but me. As the drinkers are getting drunker, louder, and sloppier, I am in control. I don't waste my time talking with anybody I don't want to deal with, I can drive anywhere and anytime I want to go, and I have a tranquility about me while I'm out and about knowing I don't have to worry about driving home. I also know I won't be waking up with a hangover.

Number 39 Be a Participant, Not a Spectator

The title comes from an experience many years ago in Tampa, Florida. I worked for a real estate developer who owned a bank in Tampa. We were in town the day before the Super Bowl was being played in Miami. Somebody asked my then-boss if he was going to the Super Bowl. This person was wealthy and had his own airplane. He could have flown across the state and spent however much cash was needed to buy a ticket. He was going to the game and was immediate with his answer. "In this life I'm a participant and not a spectator." It is a quote I have used 1,000 times in 100 different ways.

Even though I am a participant in life I have "spectated" some amazing bad television. I have watched ridiculous shows such as *Married at First Sight, 60 Days In, Work Out New York* and others. MAFS may be the dumbest. Three couples are matched. The moment they meet, they get married. A panel of "experts" reviews each person's background, upbringing, appearance, life philosophy, etc. before matching them. The premise is silly and the outcomes are sillier. Everything about this show flies in the face of evolution, attraction, and human behavior. But yet I watched. As I say about all the time I wasted being a "musclehead" at Bally's Gym: I wish I could have that time back. Same thing for MAFS. *(Confession: on occasion I've gone on the internet to find out what happened to some of the show members. I still feel bad for what Davina did to Sean on the reunion show!)*

When I was growing up, we had a Zenith television set in the living room. There were four channels, including the public television station. There was no such thing as remote control. If you wanted to change the channel, you had to walk to the set and manually turn the dial (what does that sound like to a young person?) I always joked that my skills as a wrestler were developed because of the matches I would get into with my brother over control of what we would watch.

TV has never been better than it is now. There are too many networks and too much television. Andy Warhol once said, "In the future, everybody will be famous for fifteen minutes." With the advent of hundreds of channels, reality shows on those channels, and the lower production costs, Warhol's quote may come to fruition.

You have to find ways to get away from the screen and put activity in your life. Excessive television is an assault on your impulses through the commercials and the mindless watching of shows like MAFS. If you are eating while watching TV, your concentration will be on the show you are watching and not on the food you are consuming which is a perfect prescription for overeating. Singer/actress Bette Midler once said, "Never watch anything on television dumber than you." I've spent hours and hours watching television dumber than I was or am. And I'm sure I ate tons of calories I wasn't thinking about during those wasted hours.

You need to realize that being a spectator in America usually involves food. Less spectating and more participation will result in fewer calories consumed.

Number 40 "Someday Never Comes"
I am a major fan of John Fogerty. One of the greatest singer/songwriters of all time. Whether with Creedence Clearwater Revival or on his own, his body of work has few peers.

One of my favorite songs of Fogerty's is "Someday Never Comes." It makes this list because (a) it is a great song and (b) the message is of extreme importance to this document. I knew what Number 40 was for this list before I knew what Number 1 was going to be.

I know many people who say, "Ken, someday I'm going to get a passport and start traveling like you do," or "Ken, someday I'm going to get a nice bike and go on long bike rides and climb hills like you do," or "Someday I'm going to write a book, Ken. Just like you did." And, for these folks and most others, Someday Never Comes.

If you want to start eating right and being involved in an effective and efficient exercise program (which, to reiterate, has little to do with having a gym membership), TODAY IS THE DAY TO START. Don't start following the suggestions on calorie counting "someday," do it this day.

If you're reading this and telling yourself you can't eat right, or increase your physical activity, or devote energy to creative endeavors because you don't have the time, you need to stop wasting time and make yourself more productive. We all have the same amount of minutes, hours and days. Use them wisely. There are things we all do that result in lost time. One of them, watching the local news, is something I don't do. Watching the local news is a waste of your valuable time. Identify your time wasters and convert them to productive/creative time periods. (I know I pick on the local news but the same concept applies to video games, Netflix, YouTube, DVDs, OnDemand, etc.)

A personal story that applies to this section: As detailed in Prologue Two, I've seen 36 of the 37 paintings attributed to the Dutch artist Johannes Vermeer. I saw my final Vermeer at the National Gallery in Edinburgh, Scotland. That trip included a private showing of a Vermeer owned by the Queen of England inside Buckingham Palace. When I saw my final Vermeer, a young museum docent named Rachel asked me about my Vermeer journey. She had an interest in his works. She developed her interest because she saw "Christ in the House of Mary and Martha" (Vermeer's largest painting) every working day. Rachel called over an American tourist thinking I would like to share my story. The woman was in her upper 70s, slightly bent over, walked with a cane, and had a look of constant constipation on her face. She was from Iowa. When Rachel shared with her that I had just seen my final Vermeer, the woman remarked that it was a good thing that they *("They" is everywhere*) had just found a Vermeer in somebody's attic. I explained to the woman that if a Vermeer had been found in an attic it would be international news and that I certainly would know about it. She had to tell me that she and her husband, Walter, were watching the news together and saw the story. I told her I had more than a little bit of knowledge about Vermeer and would have heard if "The Concert" was recovered. Instead of believing me, she had to call Walter over. He had the same look on his face and also walked with a cane. In Edinburgh, Scotland, two cranky people from Iowa were trying to tell me that a Vermeer painting had been found in an attic. What should have been a happy occasion for me was marred by these two curmudgeons.

Why did I share the story of Walter and his wife? When they were younger and less mean, they probably told themselves that they would go to Scotland *"someday."* They did make it, but "someday" was a little too late for them and, unfortunately, for me.

If you want to travel, write, start a business, start a biking/fitness program, start eating healthy (which this document has now defined), or devote your time and resources to a worthwhile charity, do it today and not someday—because Someday Never Comes.

Today is tomorrow yesterday. Get your stuff done—before you end up as a curmudgeonly tourist in a museum in Edinburgh, Scotland.

"Knowledge is the food of the soul."
-- Plato

EPILOGUE ONE

Equal in importance to the list of 40 ways for you to cut calories and implement them into your daily life, is the importance of understanding the significance of the Nutrition Advice Industry (NAI). The NAI (my term) is the collection of health insurance companies, government agencies, non-profit entities and, to a limited extent, the private sector that provides nutrition messages to you. Think of the amount of money spent annually by these groups to educate the masses about nutrition. I have no idea what the sum is—it could never be accurately determined—so let's just call it "a lot."

I had an insightful experience shortly after my return to the nutrition trade. I couldn't arrange seminars at the places I wanted to be because the nutritionists and "health experts" employed by these venues, instead of spending at least a few moments to determine if I had something of value to offer, joined together to prevent free of charge "Cut Your Calories...Now!!" seminars from taking place. God forbid that somebody hear about different ways to cut calories. One could only hope that these small group of nutritionists and "health experts" are as diligent with their job duties as they were in blocking my effort to do free seminars.

Here's my insight: much of the money spent on nutrition advice in our country (the country with the highest level of obesity *ever*) ends up in the pockets of Registered Dietitians (RDs) and the entities that employ them. RDs are employed by health insurers, government agencies, non-profits (American Heart Association, American Diabetes Association, et. al.), and private sector companies. The group that registers nutritionists is the Commission on Dietetic

Registration. There is a coincidental correlation between the increase in obesity and Type II diabetes (often linked to obesity) and the number of registered dietitians. The number of RDs increased by 35.4% between the years 2000 and 2014. Of course, any statistics professor would jump in here and let you know that "Correlation does not imply causation" but I default to another expression: "Where there's smoke there's fire."

Many RDs belong to a money-generating trade group called the Academy of Nutrition and Dietetics (AND). Of all the trade groups I've researched or obtained information from, this is the most profit-oriented. AND receives money from the food industry each year, and, at certain times, other sums in return for endorsements of certain food products. They accepted money once from Kellogg's to give a seal of approval for Fruit Loops as a healthy breakfast cereal. Kraft Foods (now a division of Kraft Heinz) received the "Kids Eat Right" seal for their individually wrapped cheese product from AND. This prompted Jon Stewart, formerly of *The Daily Report.* to comment on one of his shows "...this Academy is an Academy in the same way this (holding up a wrapped slice of cheese) is cheese." The past president of the group was a torch bearer for the 2012 Olympics in London. How did he get there? Coca-Cola paid for him to be there.

During my research I obtained recruiting inform-ation from AND. The material encourages RDs to join AND because there is money to be made due to "...the nation's obesity epidemic, coupled with increases in avoidable diseases and conditions such as hypertension, cardiovascular disease and diabetes..." The document neglects to state that RDs have been delivering the nation's nutrition education while all the diseases mentioned increased.

An interesting thing happened to me while trying

to return to the trade. Michael Moss, author of the immediate classic, *Salt Sugar Fat: How the Food Giants Hooked Us,* was coming to Pittsburgh to receive the Porter Prize, an annual honor awarded to an individual who advances the cause of disease prevention. I read—better to say inhaled—Moss's book and had to be in the audience. The event was held in a ballroom on the campus of the University of Pittsburgh.

Also in the audience: various RDs from the health insurance and non-profit groups in Pittsburgh. Michael Moss wrote a great book about nutrition— without being a nutritionist. Before a 2009 article on an E. coli contamination in the meat industry, Mr. Moss achieved journalistic fame for his articles related to military issues and nursing home care. Mr. Moss, while not a Registered Dietitian, had three things necessary to write the book he did: excellent and objective research skills, a sincere interest in the subject, and the ability to convey his findings to others. While Mr. Moss was discussing his work in the nutrition trade, I was waiting for at least one of the RDs in attendance to stand and ask him to get off the stage. After all, what business did he have to write about nutrition? He wasn't one of them. He wasn't an RD and wasn't a member of the Academy of Nutrition and Dietetics.

But no RD stood up.

Connected to Mr. Moss, and deserving of more attention than I can give her, is Deborah A. Cohen, MD, MPH. Dr. Cohen did us all a great favor by writing and publishing a book titled, *A Big Fat Crisis: The Hidden Forces Behind the Obesity Epidemic—And How We Can End It.* The only issue with this great book was its timing. Michael Moss's book came out before Dr. Cohen's, grabbed a tremendous amount of attention, and kept it. The book Moss wrote is great but Dr. Cohen's is equally great. Her book deserves your attention and the attention of the NAI.

The information in my list about the growth of the restaurant industry was found in her book. The concept of "product extension" (did you know there are over 60 ways to buy Oreo-related products?) is detailed in Dr. Cohen's book (an important item that the NAI neglects to share).

While reading Dr. Cohen's book, a better way for nutrition to be taught dawned on me. I have clients who have children and grandchildren with an interest in the science of food. I tell them they have to go beyond studying carbohydrates, fats, and protein and study the way food companies influence our food decisions. Find out which food companies spend the most money on TV advertising and which companies make the most financial contributions to politicians and political action committees. This is the type of information that will have value and, at this point in time, is not being provided by the RDs. We don't need more of the same. We need RDs that can make a difference.

If you are motivated after reading my book to read another book about nutrition, I would suggest Dr. Cohen's book.

EPILOGUE TWO

"The most intolerable people are provincial celebrities."
                                                --Anton Chekov

How does a quote from a Russian playwright end up in a book about my adventures in the nutrition trade? Here's how: I had been on the public service hour of a local radio station two times discussing nutrition. The shows were taped on Thursday and aired Sunday morning at 6:00 a.m. There were no commercials. I spoke for one hour. Both times, the interviewers shared that they were going to use a recording of our interview as an audition tape to look for other jobs.

There came a time when the media started reporting on the concept that eating pasta could lead to weight gain. The publicity came about because, since we had been told to eat less fat and more carbohydrates, the country had gotten noticeably fatter. The collective finger was pointed at pasta as a possible culprit.

The producer at the radio station, who booked my previous two appearances, called and asked if I wanted to return to the station to discuss this issue. This time, I would be on at 3:00 in the afternoon and interviewed by the daytime host. For me, that was primetime. This happened to be during the month of March, which is National Nutrition Month (as designated by Jon Stewart's favorite Academy) and my appearance would be promoted as such.

I drove to the station. It was a cold, snowy day in late March. Spring was nowhere to be found yet. I had a nice conversation with the station receptionist. She remembered me from the other appearances. The producer met me in the lobby and took me to the studio where the interview would take place.

I was there by myself when the interviewer walked in. I will give zero information about this person. I gave a cheerful "hello" but was met with silence. I have the unique skill of determining early on if somebody is sincerely interested in what I'm talking about, just being polite and humoring me, or if they want nothing at all to do with me. And this situation was the third one;the worst one. I was waiting for them to discuss how we would open the interview and which directions we could take. But that didn't happen. Instead, this person looked at me and said, "What are you doing here?" The news was going to be over at 3:10 p.m. and we would be on air. That time was approaching. I quickly tried to give my back story. Then I remembered that the producer had received various articles from me. I asked the interviewer if they read those pieces. "No," was the reply. "I'm too busy." I explained I had been on this station twice before talking about nutrition and fitness, the producer was familiar with my background, and had called me to discuss the concept of pasta making Americans fat. But the interviewer didn't care.

The show started. Unlike a prepared, professional host, this one gave me no slack. Their demeanor was awful. It was a nightmare. We struggled to get to the first commercial break.

Immediately at commercial, before I could ask the interviewer why they were giving me such a hard time, they picked up a telephone and made a call. I pulled some articles from my briefcase and slid them across the desk. When they got off the phone, I made a suggestion of what we could be talking about. Their reply? They ignored me.

The "On Air" light came back on. More struggle. More unfriendly, unrelated questions. I tried to engage this person in a relevant, nutrition-related on-air conversation. Nothing was working. This appearance was an embarrassing nightmare.

After the second commercial break, at about 3:25 p.m., the nightmare ended. The interviewer asked a question and I answered. They paused. And then the interviewer said, "You know, I'm getting sick and tired of everybody thinking they have the right to tell others how and what to eat." The door was open. I ran in. "Yes, (their name). I agree. And that's exactly why I'm here. I'm here to help people stop wasting time and money on nutrition and fitness products that just don't work." And then I asked, "How much money did you spend last year on weight loss products that didn't work?"

That was it. The interviewer was shooting darts at me with their eyes. If looks could kill. I held my ground. I didn't blink. The "On Air" light was still on. The interviewer looked to the phone. There were callers.

I recognized the first caller by his voice. We worked out at the same gym. He had a distinct voice, articulate with a slight accent. He probably didn't know it was me he had been listening to in this horrible interviewer with the "star" host of the station. Not everybody knew I was involved in the arena of nutrition and fitness. The caller's name was Mike. He went on to talk about how many people are inefficient in the gym and waste a lot of time there. As unfriendly as the interviewer was to me, they acted like Mike was their long lost friend. Another caller was waiting. They talked about the conflicting nature of nutrition advice and was glad to hear somebody on the radio—me—talking about the financial incentive behind nutrition advice. The callers were on my side. The interviewer started asking relevant questions and sharing personal experiences that were connected to the conversation. Their demeanor at the end of the show was 180 degrees different from the beginning.

The next week, I happened to have the radio on and tuned to this station. The interviewer announced that they had an actual nutritionist on and were going to be able to have an intelligent discussion about nutrition.

I changed the station.

Now, I know what happened to that provincial celebrity. Their career has long been over. I have no interest in talking with them. But I would like to talk to the nutritionist who was on the show the week after my appearance. I'm sure she is a member of the Academy of Nutrition and Dietetics, has gone to conferences with hotel rooms, meals, and alcohol subsidized by members of the food industry, and, when asked, has given neutral nutrition advice that wouldn't get any members of the food industry (a.k.a. possible employers) upset with her. Where is she?

Maybe she is now working for one of the food companies. If you know her—or if you are her— please contact me. I want to see what she (or you) has been doing to add to the quality of nutrition education. I also want to learn the insightful ways you've found to teach others about nutrition while the level of childhood and adult obesity has increased, while daily calorie consumption for the average American has increased, and while the food industry has increased in both size and power. And I want to read your book.

So come and find me.

Ken Kaszak
Pittsburgh, Pennsylvania
February 2019

AFTERWORD

As with most books, there are short comments (or "blurbs") on the back cover of this one. Some people contributed comments that weren't used. I already thanked all who contributed but am thanking them again with these words.

Inversely, there were people whose work was part of my learning curve who I contacted for a review of the book. Some of them are mentioned in the text. Due to their schedules, position in the Nutrition Advice Industry, or the fact they had no idea who I was or what my background is, declined the invitation to review the manuscript. And I have no issue with that. In fact, I have ongoing email correspondence with some of them.

But you—somebody who needs to start reinforcing the nutrition education presented here—should learn about the works of the individuals listed below. This part of the book is going to be your homework assignment. I want you to research the following names and determine what they contributed to nutrition education and how they helped me to advance on the learning curve of nutrition and the food industry.

Here are the names (listed alphabetically):

Steven Barrett, MD

Harriet Brown (her book, *Body of Truth*, is a must read)

T.L. (Peter) Cleave, MD

Deborah A. Cohen, MD, MPH

Gina Kolata

Robert Lustig, MD

Michael Moss

Paul Offit, MD

J. Eric Oliver, PhD
Gary Taubes
Nina Teicholz
John Yudkin, FRSC

Your assignment is to spend an uninterrupted ninety minutes on the internet to research who these people are (or were) and what their contributions to nutrition education have been. Those contributions should be taught by ever Registered Dietitian (but don't wait for that one).

I am going to close with a unique story. The leading nutrition educator and author in the world is Marion Nestle, PhD. Dr. Nestle is a professor at NYU, publishes a highly acclaimed blog, "Food Politics" (that you should be reading daily), the author of a book with the same title, and the author of numerous other books. Her reports on food studies financed by food companies should be required reading for all nutrition students.

Dr. Nestle (pronounced "Nest-el" and not like the food company) wrote a series of blogs during her trip to Cuba. She focused on agricultural issues on the island. Because I had been to Cuba many times, I had my own insight to the food situation there. I sent an email to Dr. Nestle and she replied with a short, crisp, polite reply.

I did ask her to review my manuscript. She shared that she maintains a full teaching and writing schedule and is asked to review every book about nutrition. She politely declined.

But things changed. There were blogs she wrote that had direct correlation to something that was in the first draft of this manuscript. Other blogs dealt with the stock prices of publicly-traded food manufacturers. I started to respond to those blogs and received prompt replies. I like to think that Dr. Nestle realized there was value in a person with strong research skills and no vested interest making an objective study of nutrition and nutrition education.

She agreed to review my book—on the condition it was not a diet or weight loss book (you've just read it;you know that's not the case). She was teaching in Australia and supplied me with a mailing address "down under." I sent a copy of the work to her. Weeks later I sent a follow-up message and she replied that she wouldn't be able to review the manuscript after all.

On one of my trips to Cuba, I took a beautiful photo of a small food market. The camera angle captured the yuca, "callabaza" (squash), "boniata" (sweet potatoes), "cebollas" (onions), and "frijoles y arroz" (beans and rice) on display and for sale. The food market was smaller than the average U.S. kitchen. As you've just read the book you may remember No. 34 in the 40 ways to cut calories is titled "Surround Yourself with Visions of Healthy Food." That section details my framed photo of various onion types. I made an 8 X 10 print of the Cuban food market photo and had it professionally matted and framed. I sent it to Dr. Nestle.

Her "thank you" came immediately. She further explained that the reason she didn't review this book was that is was misplaced in Australia. She went on to share that she had been thinking of hanging framed photos of healthy food scenes on her office walls. My Cuba photo was going up on the wall— just as it went up in my kitchen beneath the onion photo.

There is no comment on the back cover from Marion Nestle but she does look at the same healthy food scene I do each day. And you should be looking at the same thing—or something similar.

KK

"Nothing would be more tiresome than eating and drinking if God had not made them a pleasure as well as a necessity."

-- Voltaire

Also by Ken Kaszak:

How the Investment Business Really Works

Articles/essays available at:

www.valuekaszak.com

As Matthew Hawkins (pen name):

Under a Cuban Sky

Under a Cuban Sky, Part Two

The Confusing Muse

www.ingramcontent.com/pod-product-compliance
Lightning Source LLC
Chambersburg PA
CBHW072204280526
45788CB00002B/868